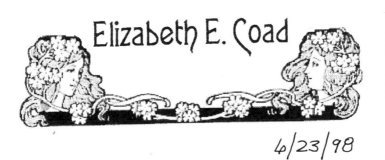

Elizabeth E. Coad

4/23/98

THE DIABETES EYE CARE SOURCEBOOK

BY

DONALD S. FONG, M.D., M.P.H. &
ROBIN DEMI ROSS, M.D.

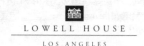

LOWELL HOUSE

LOS ANGELES

CONTEMPORY BOOKS

CHICAGO

Figures 3.1, 3.3, 3.4, 4.1, and 5.1–5.4 are reprinted with permission of the American Academy of Ophthalmology, Diabetic Retinopathy; from "The Aging Eye: Slide-Script Programs," San Francisco, 1992–1993.

Library of Congress Cataloging-in-Publication Data

Fong, Donald S.
    The diabetes eye care sourcebook / by Donald S. Fong & Robin Demi
Ross.
      p. cm.
    Includes index.
    ISBN 1-56565-875-2
    1. Diabetic retinopathy—Popular works. 2. Diabetic retinopathy—
Miscellanea. I. Ross, Robin Demi. II. Title.
RE661.D5F66 1998
617.7'3—dc21   98-9903
                                      CIP

Requests for such permissions should be addressed to:
Lowell House
2020 Avenue of the Stars, Suite 300
Los Angeles, CA 90067

Lowell House books can be purchased at special discounts when ordered in bulk for premiums and special sales.

Publisher: Jack Artenstein
Associate Publisher, Lowell House Adult: Bud Sperry
Managing Editor: Maria Magallanes
Text design: Carolyn Wendt

Manufactured in the United States of America
10 9 8 7 6 5 4 3 2 1

To my wife, Cheryl, and our daughter, Julia.

—Donald Fong

To all my great teachers and mentors who provided patient guidance, encouragement, and direction along my career path—Stanley Chang; Ravi Thomas and the Schell Eye Hospital in Vellore, South India; Tom Weingeist, Hansjoerg Kolder, Alan Kimura, Jim Folk, and the staff at the University of Iowa Hospitals and Clinics; Tom Farrell; Patty Erreto; George Williams, Mike Trese, and the entire staff of Associated Retinal Consultants in Royal Oak, Michigan; and especially my parents, Lawrence and Lorraine, and my grandparents, Henry and Matra Ross, without whom I would not have begun walking down that God-given path itself.

—Robin Demi Ross

ACKNOWLEDGMENTS

Special thanks to the American Academy of Ophthalmology for permission to use their illustrations and to Dr. Richard Brilliant, O.D., senior low-vision practitioner and associate professor at William Feinbloom Vision Rehabilitation Center, Philadelphia, Pennsylvania, for assistance with and suggestions for the low vision section and production of the low vision slides.

The authors' proceeds from this book will be channeled to diabetic retinopathy screening projects in underserved areas in the United States and the Schell Eye Hospital in Southern India.

CONTENTS

1

Types of Diabetes

We don't know exactly why people get diabetes. Sometimes it is inherited; other times it is not. Research into diabetes is ongoing, and scientists hope to develop a cure. For now, it remains a lifelong disease which requires daily attention. Our goal is to educate people about diabetes, and especially about how diabetes affects the eyes. For most people, complications from diabetes are preventable with proper screening and patient education.

It is heartbreaking to see young adults in their early twenties and thirties who come to our offices with diabetes severely affecting their eyes who have never had a previous eye examination. We know that their eye disease may have been preventable with proper early screening. Despite our best educational efforts, we still see patients, old and young, who have fallen through the cracks. Again and again, we see poor education about diabetes going hand in hand with neglect of the disease. People just don't know any better. They don't know where to get help, how to adjust their diets, what kind of exercise program they need, and what they should do to minimize complications such as blindness, kidney failure, and damage to the nerves of the hands and feet. Often, young people with diabetic complications are beginning their careers and families. They worry about losing their jobs and not being able to support their families. Parents of diabetics struggle with the problem of protecting their children while allowing them to develop independence in managing their diabetes. Because we want the best for our friends and loved ones, it is tempting to tell them what they can and cannot do. However, policing their routine will only provoke anger and contribute to lowered self-esteem. We can help them gather information and provide encouragement, but they are ultimately the ones who must live with their disease. Helping them set realistic goals that they can live with is a major focus of diabetes management.

What is diabetes?

Diabetes is a disorder of metabolism, the way our bodies use digested food for energy and growth. Most of the food we eat is broken down in the stomach and intestines by digestive juices into the simple sugar, glucose. Glucose is the body's main fuel. Glucose then passes from our stomach and intestines into our blood where it is available for body cells to use as energy. To move from the blood into our cells, insulin, a hormone produced by the pancreas, must be present. The pancreas is supposed to produce the right amount of insulin to move glucose into our cells. In diabetes, either the pancreas does not produce the right amount of insulin or the body's cells do not respond to the insulin that is produced. As a result, glucose builds up in the blood, overflows into the urine, and passes out of the body. Elevated glucose in the blood is called hyperglycemia (*hyper*—too much, *glyc*—glucose, *emia*—blood). Hyperglycemia can make you feel sick. High blood glucose over a prolonged period of time can cause damage to the blood vessels, particularly of the eyes, kidneys, and nerves. It can also worsen heart disease, cause high blood pressure, and lead to stroke.

I have heard that there are different types of diabetes and that diabetes isn't the same in everybody. What are the types of diabetes?

There are two types of diabetes. Both types cause problems with insulin and blood sugar. Insulin dependent diabetes mellitus (IDDM) is called Type I and non-insulin dependent diabetes mellitus (NIDDM) is called Type II. They differ in the age of onset, risk of diabetic ketoacidosis (diabetic coma), and method of treatment.

Type I diabetes accounts for 5 to 10 percent of all diabetes. Before developing Type I diabetes, the body made plenty of insulin; now the body has stopped making insulin. Type I diabetes is a form that commonly develops in people less than thirty years of age. All patients require insulin to prevent diabetic ketoacidosis, or diabetic coma, which can be life threatening if not recognized and treated.

In Type I diabetes, the body changes food into sugar and sends it into the blood. However, it doesn't make the necessary insulin to move the sugar into the cells. The cells don't get enough sugar and can't make energy. The cells effectively starve without the insulin to bring the sugar to them.

Type II, or NIDDM, is more common than Type I and usually begins in middle age, beyond age forty-five, but can occur earlier or later in life. Obesity is present in 60 to 80 percent of patients with Type II. It has long been considered a disease of older adults. However, recent studies suggest that more children are now developing this type of diabetes than ever before. Because of computers and video games, there is less emphasis on outdoor sports and activities. Children today are less active, and have more body fat than those of earlier generations.

Type II patients may be treated with a combination of weight loss, exercise, proper diet, and oral drugs (sulfonylureas), but many are best managed with insulin injections. The type of medication used depends on the individual. The term "non-insulin dependent" arises from the Type II patient's resistance to diabetic ketoacidosis. In this form of diabetes, the pancreas still produces insulin, but the body cannot use this insulin effectively. In spite of the presence of adequate amounts of insulin, the blood sugar levels are not normal. This type accounts for 90 to 95 percent of all diagnosed cases of diabetes.

There are two less common types of diabetes: gestational diabetes (GDM) and secondary diabetes. Gestational diabetes is diabetes which develops during pregnancy. Secondary diabetes is diabetes that is a result of medication or another disease process.

Gestational diabetes occurs during pregnancy and usually disappears after the birth of the baby. Gestational diabetes arises in about 3 percent of pregnancies. While it often wanes after delivery, women diagnosed with GDM are at increased risk for developing diabetes at a later date. GDM symptoms are usually mild and not life threatening to the woman. However, hyperglycemia, or high blood sugar, can be associated with increased problems for the baby; therefore, maintaining normal glucose levels is important during pregnancy. Obstetrician/gynecologists routinely test for glucose during pregnancy and, if necessary, run additional tests to see how the mother adjusts to being given extra sugar.

Secondary diabetes can occur with steroid use, and with diseases such as Cushing's syndrome, cystic fibrosis, and pancreatic insufficiency, which tend to increase steroid levels or damage the pancreas. Steroids are hormones that have the opposite effect from insulin. Instead of causing extra sugar to move from the bloodstream into cells, they cause sugar to increase in the bloodstream. Diseases which damage the pancreas cause the pancreas to produce little or no insulin. Alcohol can lead to inflammation of the pancreas, or pancreatitis, and diabetes.

Glucose intolerance, or borderline diabetes, is not considered a type of diabetes. When large amounts of carbohydrates are eaten, an abnormal insulin response occurs and the body is unable to metabolize the large carbohydrate load. These people are at an increased risk of developing diabetes, but most do not.

What causes diabetes to develop?

The pancreas is an organ inside the body located behind the stomach which normally makes the hormone insulin. The pancreas is composed of small islands called islets of Langerhans which contain cells called beta cells to distinguish them from other cells called alpha and delta cells. The beta cells secrete insulin. Insulin allows glucose to be taken up by the cells in the body to be used as energy.

In Type I diabetes, the beta cells completely fail to produce insulin. Many factors are theorized for this failure, including genetic predisposition, autoimmune activity, and viral causes. The immune system helps fight infection and rid the body of foreign, bad cells; however, in autoimmune diseases the immune system attacks good cells, like the beta cells of the pancreas which produce insulin. The immune system attacks itself. According to the viral theory, viruses attack the good beta cells and destroy them.

In Type II diabetes, the pancreas still produces insulin and the islet beta cells are intact; however, the body cannot use the insulin effectively. The body is essentially resistant to the normal effects of insulin. There is enough insulin in the blood but the cells don't recognize the insulin. Blood glucose levels are not normal.

What are the warning signs of diabetes? Are vision changes warning signs?

Blurry vision is one warning sign of Type I and II diabetes mellitus. The excess sugar in the blood enters the natural lens inside the eye, causing it to change shape. The effect of excess sugar in the lens is blurry vision. It is like wearing the wrong pair of eyeglasses. This visual change is usually temporary. Diabetes can also cause blurry vision by causing swelling in the central part of the retina, the macula. Macular edema can cause a change in refraction as well and make you more farsighted.

Other warning signs of Type I diabetes include:

❖ unusual thirst
❖ frequent urination

❖ extreme hunger
❖ sudden weight loss for no apparent reason
❖ unexplained weakness or fatigue
❖ nausea and vomiting

The same warning signs apply to Type II diabetes; however, there are a few additional symptoms:

❖ weight gain
❖ drowsiness
❖ itching of skin and genitals
❖ infections of skin and urinary tract
❖ tingling and numbness in the hands and feet
❖ slow healing of sores

How is diabetes diagnosed?

Diabetes may be diagnosed based on symptoms or routine blood screening. Your doctor may want to obtain a fasting blood sugar (see below) or perform a confirmation test called a glucose tolerance test (GTT). In this test, the patient drinks a concentrated amount of glucose. The glucose moves from the stomach into the blood. If the person has a normal amount of insulin, the glucose will move out of the blood and into the tissues, maintaining a normal blood glucose level.

Occasionally, a person develops complications like eye problems (retinopathy), kidney problems (nephropathy), or nerve damage (neuropathy) which suggest diabetes.

If you have classic symptoms, you should be tested immediately. You have diabetes if you meet one of the following criteria:

1. Classic symptoms and blood glucose ≥200 mg/dl.
2. Fasting blood glucose (eat no food and drink no beverages other than water within eight hours of testing) ≥126 mg/dl on two separate occasions (ADA new guideline, previous number was 140 mg/dl).
3. Fasting blood glucose ≥126 mg/dl, and two separate oral glucose tolerance tests with the two-hour glucose level ≥200 mg/dl following a glucose load of 75 grams dissolved in water.

How do I measure my sugar with a "fingerstick measuring device"?

A device which measures your blood sugar is called a glucometer or glucose meter. It can be purchased at your local pharmacy or diabetes center. A diabetes educator in your local hospital can help you find one. To check your sugar, wash your hands thoroughly and then prick your finger with a lancet. A drop of blood large enough to hang should be squeezed onto a test strip and the test strip inserted into a glucometer. The number can generally be read off the glucometer.

What makes my sugar go up?

Food, stress, and illness all increase your blood sugar. Certain foods which contain sugar and taste sweet make the blood glucose go up quickly. Other foods like bread, vegetables, and fruits cause sugar to rise more slowly. When the glucose level increases gradually, insulin has more of an opportunity to work.

HOWARD
"Diagnosis of diabetes"

A sixty-two-year-old man, Howard, was recently referred to me for blurry vision. When we dilated his eyes, we found that there were multiple splotches of blood scattered throughout his retina, the back lining of the eye (often affected by diabetes). When asked about diabetes symptoms, he admitted that he was always thirsty and drank at least 16 ounces an hour. He also mentioned urinating ten to sixteen times a day. He said he'd been feeling a little more tired for some time and slept twelve to sixteen hours a day whereas before he'd only needed seven to eight hours of sleep. He thought this was related to stress. We measured his sugar in our office using a fingerstick measuring device; the result was 162 mg/dl. We talked with him about the strong possibility that he had diabetes.

He was very worried that he might have diabetes and was afraid to find out. He finally admitted that his father had gone blind from diabetes. I sent him to see his family doctor for a glucose tolerance test, which was abnormal. He was started on some diabetes pills and also saw a diabetic educator through a free program sponsored by the hospital. The educator advised him about diet and how to change his lifestyle. The diabetic educator also told him about a diabetes support group. He returned feeling much better and very grateful for having received treatment.

What kind of doctor do I see if I think I have diabetes?

Any doctor with an M.D. or D.O. degree can make the diagnosis of diabetes. Insulin is a hormone and the medical field which manages hormones is called endocrinology. An endocrinologist is a medical internist who specializes in endocrinology, just as a cardiologist is an internist who specializes in diseases of the heart. Some endocrinologists who just take care of diabetes are called diabetologists. Many internists, emergency room physicians, and family practitioners are also well trained in the management of diabetes.

Are there any initial steps I can take if I am diagnosed with diabetes?

Yes, with the guidance of your doctor:
- ❖ lose weight
- ❖ increase physical activity
- ❖ watch your diet
- ❖ stop smoking
- ❖ treat high blood pressure

How many people in the U.S. have diabetes?

The World Health Organization estimates that there are between 100 and 120 million people with diabetes worldwide. In the United States, there are sixteen million people with diabetes. Eight million Americans have been diagnosed and a new case is diagnosed each minute. Another eight million have the disease but are undiagnosed Type II diabetics.

Is diabetes more common in any particular ethnic group?

Many ethnic groups, especially Native Americans, have a very high incidence of diabetes and subsequently of diabetic retinopathy. One tribe, the Puma Indians of Arizona, have a 50 percent rate of diabetes on their reservation. No ethnic group is free of diabetes whether in the United States or abroad. A concerted effort must be made to educate all people about diabetes.

Table 1.1 OCCURRENCE OF DIABETES IN ETHNIC GROUPS

Native Americans	5–50%
Caucasians	6.2%
Cuban Americans	9.1%
African Americans	9.6%
Mexican Americans	9.6%
Puerto Ricans	10.9%
Japanese Americans*	10–20%

* Japanese Americans age 45 to 74 living in King County, Washington have a 20% incidence in men and a 10% incidence in women.

Who is at risk for diabetes and should be tested frequently?

Consider testing all persons age forty-five and older (if normal, repeat every three years). Consider testing at a younger age, or more frequently, for any of the following:

❖ members of high-risk ethnic groups such as African Americans, Hispanics, and Native Americans

❖ those who are obese (more than 20 percent over desirable weight)

❖ those who have a close relative with diabetes

❖ women who have delivered a baby weighing more than 9 pounds or who have been diagnosed with gestational diabetes

❖ those with high blood pressure (140/90 millimeters of mercury or higher)

❖ those with low levels of HDL cholesterol (35 milligrams per deciliter or lower) or high triglyceride levels (250 milligrams per deciliter or higher) or both

❖ those who on previous testing had impaired glucose tolerance (140–199 mg/dl on a two-hour test) or impaired fasting glucose (110–125 mg/dl)

How does diabetes affect other diseases, such as high blood pressure? Can these other diseases affect my eyesight?

In Type II diabetes, 60 to 65 percent of all patients also have high blood pressure. In Type I diabetes, 22 percent of all patients have high blood pressure. This is significantly higher than the nondiabetic population.

Blood pressure is the force exerted by blood against blood vessel walls. Each time your heart beats, it causes a surge of pressure, which is called systolic pressure. When the heart rests between beats, the blood pressure is lower; this is called diastolic pressure. Blood pressure is represented by two numbers, such as 120/80. The upper number (120) is the systolic pressure and the lower number (80) is the diastolic pressure.

Blood pressure readings vary over the course of the day, so it is important to take more than one reading over a period of time. If blood pressure readings are consistently higher than 140/90, it usually indicates high blood pressure. It is important that diabetics have their blood pressure checked regularly.

High blood pressure can cause damage to three parts of the eye—the optic nerve, the choroid, and the retina. The choroid is the spongy layer of blood located beneath the retina. It provides nourishment to the inner two-thirds of the retina. The optic nerve is the electrical connection between the retina and the brain.

The risk of stroke in diabetics is two and a half times higher than normal and the risk of atherosclerosis of the coronary (heart) and periphery (legs and neck) is three times more common in diabetics. Atherosclerosis is the disease in which cholesterol builds up along the vessel walls of the arteries. Some people call this disease "hardening of the arteries."

Atherosclerosis and high blood pressure are both risk factors for vein and artery occlusions in the eye. The back lining of the eye, the retina, contains blood vessels that provide nourishment to the eye. These tiny blood vessels are susceptible to closure from within by clotted blood and cholesterol plaques. At other places, a "hardened artery" may pass across a vein and press on the vein from the outside. This can cause a vein occlusion, which is like someone permanently stepping on a garden hose and preventing the flow of water from the faucet to the nozzle. Dramatic vision loss can occur from a central retinal artery or central retinal vein occlusion.

Stroke affects the brain. The various parts of the brain are supplied by blood vessels. In stroke, one or more of those blood vessels stops perfusing, or supplying a particular area of the brain. Let's say that a particular part of the brain is responsible for you being able to move your right leg. If that part of the brain suddenly loses its supply of blood, your right leg may be partially or fully paralyzed, depending upon the length of time the blood supply was cut off.

Does the type of diabetes I have reflect the type of eye complication I might get?

Yes. Juvenile onset diabetes (Type I) carries a higher risk of severe proliferative retinopathy. Many studies have reported a connection between the severity of the retinopathy and the duration of the diabetes in Type I patients. In Type I diabetics, 18 percent have some form of retinopathy after three to four years of diabetes; this increases to over 80 percent after fifteen or more years. The frequency of proliferative retinopathy increases from 0 percent after four years of the disease to 25 percent after fifteen years and up to 50 percent after twenty years.

After fifteen years with the disease, 15 percent will have macula edema. Over a lifetime, 42 percent of Type I diabetics will develop macula edema and 72 percent will eventually develop proliferate diabetic retinopathy (PDR), which requires laser treatment.

The development of vision-threatening retinopathy is rare in children prior to puberty. When diabetes is diagnosed between ages ten and thirty, significant retinopathy can become apparent after six to seven years. However, because there are more adult onset (Type II) cases, Type II patients comprise a significant proportion of individuals with blinding complications like macular edema and proliferative diabetic retinopathy, as well as neovascular glaucoma.

Up to 3 percent of patients first diagnosed after age thirty have clinically significant macular edema or high-risk characteristics at the time of diagnosis of diabetes. About 50 percent have some degree of retinopathy after twenty years with the disease. Less than 10 percent of non-insulin takers develop proliferative disease.

Is treatment successful in eliminating blindness from diabetes?

No. Treatment is effective in significantly reducing, but not eliminating, the risk of visual loss from diabetic retinal disease.

The earlier a complication is detected, the more probable that further vision loss can be prevented or slowed. Unfortunately, many diabetic patients are not examined by an ophthalmologist. In one study, 55 percent of patients with a high risk of vision loss had never received laser treatment when needed. Continuing care with an ophthalmologist is very important in lowering your chance of blindness.

My primary care doctor looks in my eyes. Isn't that eye examination sufficient?

No. It is unlikely that your primary care doctor performs a dilated eye examination in his or her office. Dilation is critical for properly detecting retinopathy. Correct dilation requires the use of dilating drops. When your primary care doctor looks in your eyes, he or she uses a direct ophthalmoscope. This is a handheld instrument that allows the doctor to see your nerve, the vessels, and the macula. It provides a poor view of the peripheral retina.

Unless the retina periphery is examined, a good proportion of diabetic retinopathy will be missed. In one study, 27 percent of retinal abnormalities were found outside the central 45-degree zone. The peripheral retina is best evaluated with an indirect ophthalmoscope, which is worn on the head while viewing your retina through a special handheld lens.

When should I see an ophthalmologist for an examination?

If you are age thirty or younger, the American Academy of Ophthalmology recommends that you have an eye examination within five years of diagnosis of Type I diabetes. If you are over age thirty and have Type II diabetes, you should be seen right at the time of diagnosis. Many patients with Type II diabetes have had diabetes for many years prior to being diagnosed.

If you are considering a pregnancy and have any type of diabetes, you should be seen before you are pregnant. If you have diabetes and are pregnant, you should be seen right away and at least every three months during your pregnancy.

In addition to seeing an eye doctor regularly, what else can I do to minimize my chances of losing vision and developing complications from diabetes?

Everyone is different and adjusts differently to diabetes. Not everyone with diabetes gets the same treatment plan. It is tempting to compare your treatment plan to another diabetic's. It is tempting to disregard the guidelines established for your diabetes. Don't! Remember, your treatment plan is designed especially for you and may need to be adjusted to find your most ideal plan. Your doctor may ask you to keep a daily log of your diet and sugars to help determine how to adjust your diabetes medications.

1. Good glucose control is essential in preventing the complications of diabetes. The Diabetes Control and Complications Trial (DCCT) was a specially designed study which looked at the relationship between good glucose control and diabetic complications. It showed that blood sugar levels greater than 200 mg/dl were

associated with increased complications. (See Chapter 6 for more detailed information.)

2. Diabetes affects multiple parts of the body and regular care by a primary physician is essential. Ideally, that doctor should have a special interest in diabetes and have access to a health care team which includes diabetic educators, dietitians, social workers, and counselors. In the DCCT, the patients who lowered their risk of complications were surrounded or in contact with a health care team on a monthly basis.

3. Don't ignore the importance of managing cholesterol and blood pressure so that you don't develop additional eye problems or worsen your diabetic retinopathy.

4. See an ophthalmologist knowledgeable and experienced in the management of diabetic retinopathy. Ophthalmologists with specialized knowledge and experience may be better able to detect and treat serious disease. Patients with significant retinopathy should see a specialist. Referral may also be useful if there is uncertainty concerning the reason for decreased vision.

5. Diet and exercise are often incorporated into your treatment plan. You will need help and advice from dietitians having special knowledge about diabetes. You will also need guidance and training through the help of certified diabetic educators about how to manage your diabetes. A diabetes educator is trained to teach people about living with diabetes. He or she may be a nurse, dietitian, exercise expert, physician, or pharmacist. These experts are invaluable resources. They can help you set realistic goals that will help avoid "burnout" from unattainable ideals in diabetes management. Call your local hospital and ask for the

diabetic education team, or contact the American Association of Diabetic Educators (see Appendix C) to obtain a local listing in your area. Visits with diabetes educators are usually covered by insurance.

6. Know your rights as a patient. Investigate your health care plan thoroughly. Do you have a choice of doctors? If you have been seeing another ophthalmologist not included in your care plan, can an exception be made? Understand how a referral takes place. Your primary care doctor managing your diabetes often acts as a "gatekeeper." A gatekeeper tries to prevent unnecessary tests from being ordered. Your primary care doctor gives permission for you to be evaluated and treated by an ophthalmologist. This evaluation and treatment usually includes an eye examination, a fluorescein angiogram, color photographs of the back of your eye, and possibly laser treatment. Preventive care and education often have a low priority with some managed care companies. Check to see whether diabetic education and dietary and nutritional consultation are included, as well as low vision consultation. Know your rights!

2

Eye Problems and Diabetes

In diabetes, the body is not able to process sugar properly. Diabetes affects the brain, the heart, the digestive tract, the reproductive system, and the arms and legs. In addition to these problems, diabetes affects every part of your eye. Diabetes can lead to changes in your prescription for glasses. It can lead to glaucoma, cataracts, diabetic retinopathy, and other problems.

Refractive Error

What is refractive error?

Normally, light entering the eye passes through the cornea and lens and is focused on the center of the retina. Refractive error is an eye condition where light entering the eye cannot be focused on the retina.

What causes refractive errors?

The eye can be thought of as a camera. Just like a camera, the eye has lenses that focus light. There are two principal lenses: the cornea (the clear transparent front portion of your eye), and the lens inside the eye. However, only the inside lens is able to adjust the eye's focus to allow you to see things up close and far away. In people who do not need glasses, the power of the cornea and lens just balance out so that they focus the light precisely onto the retina (the "film" of the eye). If the light is focused in front of the retina, the person is nearsighted. If the light is focused behind the retina, the person is farsighted. Whenever the light is not focused exactly on the retina, there is a refractive error.

Diabetes can lead to changes in refractive error. These changes occur because the blood sugar level varies.

Who gets refractive errors?

Refractive errors are quite common in the United States. About 25 percent of the population is nearsighted (myopic). Most of the time, nearsightedness is due to changes in the shape of the eye. Often, nearsighted eyes are longer. The majority of people become nearsighted during school age to adolescence. Once it develops, this refractive error remains for the life of the individual.

Patients with diabetes may develop myopia during childhood. However, diabetics also can develop transient changes in their refractive errors. This is probably the most common eye problem experienced by patients with diabetes. Patients often notice changes in their vision when their blood sugar goes up. With elevated sugars in the blood, sugar is also raised in the lens. Higher sugar levels in the lens leads to swelling of the lens. This increase in size leads to changes in the refractive error of the eye.

What are the symptoms?

Blurry vision is probably the most common symptom. Blurry vision is a strong indicator that the blood sugar level may be high, and you should check your blood sugar and make the proper adjustments.

How are refractive errors diagnosed?

Because refractive errors in diabetes are often transient, correcting the high blood sugar level may be all that is necessary. Most of the time, temporary refractive errors do not need treatment. If you experience blurry vision, you should be examined by your eye doctor. He or she will check you for this condition by measuring your vision with various lenses to see whether your vision would improve.

How is refractive error treated?

Permanent refractive errors are treated by prescription glasses or contact lenses. However, glasses are not always the best solution for diabetics. Because the refractive error from diabetes may be temporary, your eye doctor may ask you to stabilize your blood sugar levels to see if the refractive error resolves. If after the blood sugar levels are stable and you still experience blurry vision, then your eye doctor may prescribe glasses. Remember that if your sugar levels vary a lot, your refractive error is also going to vary. A pair of glasses prescribed on a day when your blood sugar is at one level may not work on another day when it is at another level. Keeping clear vision is another reason to try to keep your diabetes under good control. You should not get your eyes measured for glasses if you have recently changed your control regimen. When you go to your eye doctor to be measured for glasses, you should be sure that your blood sugar levels have been stable for at least a couple of weeks.

Cataracts

What is a cataract?

The lens is the part of the eye that focuses entering light. With age and under certain conditions, the normally clear lens becomes cloudy. This cloudiness is called a cataract. A cataract can block incoming light and lead to loss of vision.

What causes a cataract?

Age is the most common cause of cataracts. Almost everyone over the age of fifty has loss of transparency in their lenses. However, not all cataracts lead to visual loss. Often a cataract can be diagnosed by your eye doctor and you may not have noticed any vision change. In these cases, the cataract is said to be "not visually impairing."

Diabetes is another common cause of cataracts. In addition to causing swelling of the lens and changes in refractive error, diabetes also can cause changes in the clarity of the lens. High blood sugar levels that last a long time can lead to cloudiness in the lens. Normally, the lens must be crystal clear for the light passing through it to be focused on the retina. The lens is comprised primarily of water and protein. The protein is arranged in a very ordered way to let light pass through. With diabetes and age, some of the protein may clump together and form a small cloudy area in the lens. These cloudy areas then distort and block vision, and may also cause double vision.

What are the symptoms of a cataract?

Cataracts can cause a variety of symptoms. Early on, a mild cataract may not lead to any symptoms. With time, as the cloudiness worsens, less light enters the eye and loss of vision might be experienced. Patients with cataracts often report that their vision is blurry, like looking through fog. Because cataracts are opacities in the lens, the cloudy areas can also lead to scattering of the light coming into the eye. This scattering of light is called glare; the patient may notice that light seems to be coming from everywhere. Glare is most bothersome on bright days, but you may also notice it at night while driving. Oncoming headlights appear like a point of light with multiple light streaks. Finally, cataracts can lead to dulling of colors.

How is a cataract diagnosed?

Although you may think you have a cataract, the only way to know for sure is to have an eye examination. Your ophthalmologist will instill some eyedrops into your eyes to dilate the pupils. He or she then will examine the lens of your eyes with the slit lamp biomicroscope.

GEROME
"Cataract surgery"

Gerome is a seventy-two-year-old man who came to me disappointed with his cataract surgery. He told me that he did not see well with his right eye. On further questioning, he informed me that he was told he needed laser treatment, but he was hesitant. When he finally decided to have it, his doctor told him that it was too late. He needed major eye surgery, but he hesitated on this as well. Since that time, he has not been able to see out of that eye at all.

I asked about his left eye. He told me that he had also needed laser treatment on the left eye but that he thought he outgrew the need for it. He was doing fine until a year ago when he noticed very gradual loss of vision in his left eye and was told a growing cataract was the reason. Convinced that the problem was a cataract, he underwent cataract surgery. His vision before the surgery was 20/50. However, after surgery, his vision did not improve and even got worse. When he did not recover vision, he came in to see me.

Gerome was not able to see anything out of his right eye, not even light. With his left eye, he was able to make out only the big "E" on the chart. After dilating his pupils, I examined the inside of his eyes. The right eye was quite scarred and I was not able to see his retina at all. On the left, the view inside was very hazy. I was able to make out a lot of scarring, bleeding inside the eye, and possibly swelling inside in the macula.

Cataract surgery in patients with diabetes is not a sure thing. Only about one-third of eyes see better and it is often only one or two lines better on the eye chart. One-third get no improvement and one-third do worse. Gerome's left eye falls into this last category. After cataract surgery in diabetics, the retinopathy can progress, there can be vitreous hemorrhage, and the macula often gets more edematous.

Because Gerome only had one eye and he was in effect legally blind after the cataract surgery, we talked about what options were available. After extensive discussion, we decided to do a vitrectomy operation to remove the blood from inside the eyes and to use the laser (remember, Gerome had no previous laser surgery). However, even after a very successful vitrectomy operation, Gerome could not see better.

Whenever a patient with diabetes wants to have cataract surgery, I always tell him this story. Cataract surgery in diabetics is just not as successful as in the general population, and the patient must understand that there are significant risks of losing vision from surgery.

When should a cataract be treated?

If your eye care professional finds a cataract, you may not need cataract surgery for several years, or for that matter, ever in your lifetime. In general, if you have decreased vision which limits your ability to perform daily activities such as reading, writing, or driving, and your doctor believes the problem is due to the cataract, then treatment may be necessary.

Although cataract surgery is very successful for patients without diabetes, the potential for excellent vision following cataract surgery for diabetics is more limited. No one is sure why diabetics do not see as well after cataract surgery, but there may be several reasons. Cataract surgery for such patients is more difficult. Leakage from the retina (macular edema) is much more common in patients with diabetes. Finally, the retina and macula in diabetics may already have sustained some damage from the diabetes. This damage likely limits the amount of good vision that can be recovered following cataract surgery.

How are cataracts treated?

Some of the cataractous changes in the eyes of diabetic patients can be transient. In fact, after correction of high blood sugars, the changes can resolve and vision may return. However, with chronic elevations in blood sugar and age, some of the changes can become permanent. At present, there is only one way to deal with these permanent cataracts. No medicine or eyedrops is effective in clearing the lenses. People often ask whether the cataract can be removed with a laser, but the only treatment available is surgical removal of the cloudy lens.

The surgery usually takes about one hour. Most of the time, cataract surgery is done on an outpatient basis. Your eye is made numb (anesthetized) with an injection before the actual eye surgery. The cloudy lens is removed and replaced with a clear plastic lens. After the surgery, you can usually go home the same day with a patch over your eye. The following day, your doctor will check the eye. If everything looks good, your doctor will ask you to use eye-drops to prevent infection (antibiotics) and to reduce the inflammation (steroids).

Glaucoma

What is glaucoma?

Glaucoma is an eye disease in which the fluid pressure in the eye is elevated, leading to damage of the optic nerve and loss of vision and possibly blindness. There are two forms of glaucoma more common in patients with diabetes: open-angle glaucoma and neovascular glaucoma.

What causes glaucoma?

Behind the cornea, in the front of the eye, there is a small fluid-filled space called the anterior chamber. Clear fluid flows into this chamber to bathe and nourish the lens. Normally, this fluid leaves the eye through a drainage network in the eye (trabecular meshwork), maintaining a normal pressure. In angle closure glaucoma, fluid produced in the eye is unable to drain out through the angle and trabecular meshwork. As the fluid builds up, the pressure inside the eye rises. Unless this pressure is controlled, it may cause damage to the optic nerve. In open-angle glaucoma, the cause of the elevated pressure is unclear. In neovascular glaucoma, new blood vessels grow over the drainage network of the eye. This blocks the drain and prevents the fluid from emptying.

Who gets glaucoma?

Patients with diabetes are twice as likely than normal to develop glaucoma. If you have diabetes and advanced retinopathy, you are at higher risk for glaucoma. In addition, African Americans over age forty, people over age sixty, and people with a family history of glaucoma are more at risk.

What are the symptoms of glaucoma?

At first, there are no symptoms. Vision stays normal and there is no pain. Glaucoma is known as a "silent thief," stealing vision without your awareness. As the disease progresses, a person with glaucoma may notice his side vision (peripheral vision) diminish gradually, even though central (straight-ahead) vision is just fine. Often, loss of peripheral vision is not noticed by the patient. As the disease worsens, more and more of a person's peripheral vision may be lost. Eventually, in untreated glaucoma, the central vision will also be lost.

How is glaucoma diagnosed?

Glaucoma is diagnosed with three procedures. The first step is to check the pressure in both eyes. The second step is to examine the optic nerve of both eyes. Your doctor will likely instill some drops into your eyes to dilate the pupils. Dilation of the pupils will allow him or her to examine the retina in addition to the optic nerve. Examination of the optic nerve will provide clues as to whether glaucoma is present. The third step involves testing your peripheral vision. This is a special test in which the patient stares at a large lighted bowl, and is asked to indicate by pressing a button whenever a light is seen coming into the peripheral vision. The visual field test takes about twenty minutes per eye; each eye is usually tested separately.

How is glaucoma treated?

At present, there is no known cure for glaucoma, but there are several treatments that can slow down its progression.

The first treatment is medication. These drugs may be either eyedrops or pills. Some eyedrops reduce the pressure in the eye by slowing the production of fluid, while others improve the drainage of the eye. The pills usually work by reducing the production of fluid. For most people, medications can control the eye pressure. However, over time, some of the medications may lose their effects. In addition, medications may cause intolerable side effects over many years or decades.

The second treatment option is laser surgery. A laser is a very strong, focused beam of light. Laser is often used at the drainage network of the eye to increase the outflow of fluid. This procedure is successful 80 percent of the time. However, over time, the effect of the laser may wear off and traditional surgery may become necessary.

The third treatment is an operation on the eye. The goal of most glaucoma surgery is to make another drainage option for the fluid inside the eye. Techniques include various ways of making a new drain.

Diabetic Retinopathy

What is retinopathy?

Diabetic retinopathy is the eye disease that develops when high blood sugar damages the blood vessels in the retina. The manifestations of these damaged blood vessels include bleeding in the retina (retinal hemorrhages), leakage of fluid (edema), and closure of blood vessels. Diabetic retinopathy is the leading cause of blindness in American adults.

The very first change that develops in diabetic retinopathy is loss of the cells lining the blood vessels in the retina. Over time, the blood vessels become weak and become leaky. Later, blood vessels close off and stop delivering blood to parts of the retina. This loss of blood flow causes part of the retina to be starved for blood. The technical term for this condition is ischemia. As this happens, abnormal new blood vessels grow into these areas to try to replenish the lost blood supply. Unfortunately, these new blood vessels (neovascularization) are not helpful and cause more problems than they solve.

Not only are these new blood vessels unable to supply the necessary blood flow, but they cause problems. These new blood vessels are very weak and are prone to bleeding. Normally, the inside of the eye, the vitreous cavity, is clear and allows light to pass through the eye to land on the retina. With blood in this normally clear space, the light is blocked and vision loss develops. Bleeding into the clear hollow part of the eye is called a vitreous hemorrhage.

Over time, these new blood vessels develop into scar tissue. Just like the scar tissue which forms from cuts on your skin, scar tissue in your eye contracts. Contracture of scar tissue is part of the normal process of healing. However, in the eye where structures are very delicate, any contracture or scar tissue formation is harmful. In eyes where there is a great deal of scar tissue, the scar tissue actually can cause a retinal detachment (separation of the retina from its nourishing layer in the eye wall). This separation of the retina from the underlying layer causes the retina to stop working and vision loss occurs.

What causes diabetic retinopathy?

Diabetic retinopathy is caused by damage to the blood vessels of the retina. We now know that high blood levels of glucose damage the cells that line the blood vessels.

Who gets diabetic retinopathy?

Anyone with diabetes can get diabetic retinopathy. The longer someone has diabetes, the more likely he or she will develop it. Nearly everyone with diabetes will eventually develop some retinopathy. Table 2.1 lists factors that increase the likelihood of developing retinopathy, especially the more severe proliferative retinopathy.

How is diabetic retinopathy diagnosed?

Diabetic retinopathy is diagnosed by examining the retina. During your examination, your ophthalmologist will instill eyedrops into your eyes to dilate your pupils. Dilated pupils allow your eye doctor to examine your retina completely. (An undilated examination does not permit a thorough examination of your retina.)

Table 2.1   FACTORS AFFECTING THE DEVELOPMENT OF RETINOPATHY

Type of diabetes

In the United States, there are two major types of diabetes: Type I and Type II (see Table 2.2). In Type I diabetes, insulin is required to prevent the development of diabetic ketoacidosis, a life-threatening complication. In Type II diabetes, insulin is helpful, but is not essential for life. Patients with Type II diabetes will not develop diabetic ketoacidosis if insulin is withheld. Patients with Type I are more likely to develop more severe retinopathy. Patients with Type II develop less severe retinopathy, but may develop macular edema more often.

Duration

The longer you have had diabetes, the more likely you will have some form of retinopathy.

Hyperglycemia

The higher your blood sugar, the more likely you will have retinopathy, especially the more severe retinopathy.

High blood pressure (Hypertension)

High blood pressure (hypertension) increases the risk of developing more severe diabetic retinopathy. Treatment of high blood pressure can prevent cardiovascular disease, stroke, and death. Hypertension itself can cause its own form of retinopathy. You might have hypertensive retinopathy as well as diabetic retinopathy.

Proteinuria and renal disease

Many studies have shown that having diabetic kidney disease also increases your risk of having retinopathy.

Table 2.1 *continued*

Gender

Although some studies have shown that there is more severe diabetic retinopathy in young adult men, the frequency of disease is probably similar between men and women.

Race

Pima Indians have the highest frequency of diabetes. Almost 80 percent of Pima Indians develop diabetes. Mexican Americans also have a high prevalence of diabetes and are thought to have more severe forms of diabetic retinopathy.

Genetics

Genetic factors probably play a role in the development of diabetic retinopathy.

Age at examination

Prior to puberty, children rarely develop diabetic retinopathy regardless of how long they have had diabetes. Numerous hormonal changes occur at puberty and probably affect the development of retinopathy.

Age at diagnosis

Most studies have shown that older persons with diabetes are more likely to have some diabetic retinopathy. However, it is the younger patients with diabetes that have the more severe form of the illness.

Body weight

Although obesity increases the risk of developing diabetes, it does not seem to increase the risk of developing retinopathy or of developing more severe retinopathy.

continued

Table 2.1 *continued*

Lipids

High cholesterol is harmful to all blood vessels in the body. It increases the risk of heart disease and stroke and increases the risk of death. In the eye, high cholesterol can lead to vision loss. Cholesterol deposits can develop in the retina and lead to visual loss.

Pregnancy

Pregnancy increases the risk of developing more severe retinopathy.

Smoking

Although smoking has never been shown to worsen retinopathy, smoking increases the risk of heart attacks, strokes, and death. If you have "dry" macular degeneration, smoking increases your risk of developing "wet" macular degeneration. The "wet" form of macular degeneration is another cause of blindness among elderly patients.

Aspirin use

Aspirin has not been shown to have any significant effect on diabetic retinopathy or cataracts.

Alcohol

Alcohol can be metabolized by the body into sugar, which then elevates the blood sugar levels. However, alcohol is not a substitute for food and can cause dehydration. In addition, consumption of large amounts of alcohol can damage the optic nerve by lowering the level of essential vitamins such as vitamin B_{12} and thiamine.

Table 2.2 TYPES OF DIABETES

Type	Characteristics
Type I Insulin Dependent Diabetes Mellitus (IDDM)	Affects younger patients Insulin necessary to prevent development of diabetic ketoacidosis
Type II Non-Insulin Dependent Diabetes Mellitus (NIDDM)	Affects older patients Insulin not necessary to prevent development of diabetic ketoacidosis

When your eye doctor examines your retina, he or she will determine the level of retinopathy in your eyes and whether your eyes have leakage in the center of the retina. Retinopathy is divided into two types, depending on the presence of new blood vessels (neovascularization) growing on the retinal surface (see Table 2.3). The type with neovascularization is called proliferative diabetic retinopathy (PDR), and the types without it are called nonproliferative diabetic retinopathy (NPDR). PDR entails a high chance of visual loss and often requires laser treatment without delay. NPDR is often divided into mild, moderate, and severe forms. The severity of NPDR is graded on the probability of developing neovascularization.

In addition to checking the level of retinopathy, your eye doctor also will determine whether there is leakage in the center of the macula (macular edema). If macular edema is present, he or she will determine whether it is clinically significant. Clinically significant macular edema (CSME) may require laser treatment.

Table 2.3   LEVELS OF RETINOPATHY AND THEIR RISKS

Type of Retinopathy	Risks
Mild NPDR*	Low severity Low risk for visual loss ± Macular edema
Moderate NPDR	± Macular edema
Severe NPDR	± Macular edema
Mild PDR**	± Macular edema
High risk PDR	Very severe retinopathy High risk for visual loss ± Macular edema

* Nonproliferative Diabetic Retinopathy.
** Proliferative Diabetic Retinopathy.
± Macular edema can develop at each level of retinopathy. Its presence increases the risk of visual loss.

What are the symptoms of retinopathy?

There are often no symptoms until late in the disease. Vision may not change until the problem is quite advanced, when loss of vision could be quite sudden. There is usually no pain. Discomfort may be due to problems other than diabetic retinopathy.

Blurred vision can be a sign of edema or hemorrhage. The most sensitive portion of your retina is called the macula. Swelling of the macula can lead to diminished vision. In addition, bleeding into the vitreous can also lead to decreased vision. The important thing to remember is that the disease may progress a great deal before you experience any symptoms.

As with any disease, diabetic retinopathy is easier to treat if diagnosed early. The only way to prevent its progression is to have regular eye examinations.

How is retinopathy treated?

At present, there are no eyedrops or pills that can treat diabetic retinopathy. The early forms of the disease are treated with laser, and the more severe forms often require major surgery (see Chapters 4 and 5 on the treatment of diabetic retinopathy).

3

Eye Examinations and Diabetes

Years ago, a Gallup poll of Americans, both with and without diabetes, showed that blindness and cancer were the two medical conditions people feared most. Although diabetic retinopathy is the leading cause of new cases of blindness each year, less than half of all diabetics get a yearly eye examination. Diabetes is a lifelong disease requiring many adjustments. These adjustments include diet, exercise, medications, doctor's visits, and sometimes testing to help minimize problems related to the diabetes. Because diabetes can affect the eyes, kidneys, and nerves, the eye examination is a very important part of the health care for every diabetic.

Despite their knowledge of its importance, only 40 percent of all diabetics get a vision screening examination. Many people are afraid to have their eyes examined because they are afraid of bad news if they report their blurry vision. Other people rationalize that if they had eye problems related to their diabetes, their vision would be blurry, so they don't need an eye examination.

No one knows exactly how diabetes causes damage to the eyes, but one fact is indisputable: people with diabetes are at an increased risk for blindness. The longer someone has had the disease, the greater the risk. Fortunately, medical progress has made it possible to *prevent and minimize* damage to the eyes caused by diabetes with early diagnosis and treatment.

Realizing the importance of the eye examination in preventing vision loss from diabetes is crucial. Vision can be perfect, yet diabetes can damage the eye. Understanding the anatomy or the parts of the eye can help you comprehend the many parts of the eye examination. This can make the visit to the eye doctor less frightening. Knowledge is one step toward taking control of your diabetes rather than letting it control you. Remember, knowledge is power!

Basic Anatomy of the Eye

What are the different parts of the eye? How does the eye work?

To understand how diabetes can damage the eye, it is important to know how the healthy eye works. The eye is located within a bony protective cone called the orbit. The orbit is shaped like a pointed ice cream cone and has fragile walls which are susceptible to fracture when an injury occurs. The sinuses surround the orbits and are located within the skull. Sinuses are basically boxes of air that connect to the nasal passages.

The eye itself is shaped like a ball. The tough outer covering is called the sclera, and the sclera protects the delicate structures inside which are responsible for vision. There is a thin membrane which covers the sclera called the conjunctiva. The conjunctiva contains the blood vessels on the covering of the eye. If you rub your eye, these vessels become visible and the eye may appear red.

The sclera is often called the "white of the eye." The sclera envelops the majority of the eye except the front cover, which is crystal clear like a car's windshield. This crystal-clear area is called the cornea, and it is curved (see Figure 3.1). The cornea is very sensitive and has many fine nerves which innervate it or stimulate it. When a person gets a scratch on the cornea's surface, this "cornea-abrasion" can be very painful and require medical attention.

Light enters the eye through the clear cornea and passes

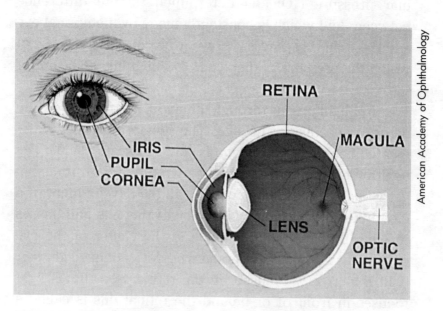

Figure 3.1 Schematic of the eye

through a liquid space called the anterior chamber, then through the pupil, or diaphragm of the eye. The pupil is the round hole in the iris. The iris is the colored part of the eye. Like a camera diaphragm, the pupil regulates the amount of light entering the eye. When a bright light enters the eye through the pupil, the pupil gets smaller or constricts. When it is dark, the pupil dilates or gets bigger to let in more light.

The angle of the eye is the angle where the cornea meets the iris. The space between is referred to as the drainage angle, where the fluid leaves the eye. The eye maintains a pressure, called the intraocular pressure, so that the eye does not deflate like a flat tire. The normal pressure in the eye is between 10 and 21 millimeters of mercury (like the weatherman's barometric scale) and can vary within this normal range over the course of the day, with the peak pressure in the eye often occurring in the early morning hours. Intraocular pressure (IOP) is determined by the difference between fluid which is constantly made by the normal eye and the fluid that leaves the eye. Glaucoma is a disease in which the pressure in the eye is too high for the health of the optic nerve.

After light passes through the pupil, it is focused by the natural lens inside the eye. The lens within the eye is located behind the pupil and is shaped like an M&M®. The healthy lens is clear like plastic wrap, but with time can get cloudy like wax paper. (We call the development of a cloudy lens a cataract.) Light leaves the lens and passes through the jellylike substance in the center of the eye called the vitreous. In a person who does not need glasses, light is perfectly focused on the retina. Sometimes light focuses in front of or behind the retina; this is called a refractive error and requires corrective lenses. Your glasses or contact lens prescription provides the precise correction and allows light to focus sharply on the retina so that images are clear.

The retina acts like the film in a camera and records the images focused on it. There are multiple layers within the retina. These layers contain fine electrical connections and circuits which ultimately connect to the brain. The retina also contains blood vessels, which deliver the necessary nutrients to the retina to keep it healthy. The retina contains both arteries and veins. The arteries originate from the heart and the major arteries in the neck, then travel through the optic nerve to enter the retina. Here, they become thinner and tinier and are called arterioles. They supply nutrients and oxygen to the retina. Deoxygenated blood (blood without oxygen) then travels back through veins to the vessels in the neck and back to the heart and lungs to become oxygenated again so the cycle can be repeated.

Just as your arm has different parts (elbow, wrist, hand), so the retina is composed of different parts. You have two types of vision: central vision and peripheral vision. Central vision allows you to see people's faces and read letters, while peripheral (side) vision lets you see a car moving beside you while your eyes stay focused straight ahead on the road. The macula is the center section of the retina and is responsible for your central vision.

Unlike the film in a camera, the light on the retina is converted to electrical impulses, which are collectively sent to the brain via the optic nerve. The optic nerve looks like a cord which exits the back of the eye and travels through the orbit to connect with the brain, the main electric warehouse.

JOYCE
"Overcoming eye examination fears"

One of my favorite patients, Joyce, is a sixty-three-year-old woman who works as a dishwasher in a local hospital. Joyce had never had her eyes dilated despite having had diabetes for twenty-six years. Joyce confided from the start that she was afraid of going blind. Her son explained that he strongly encouraged his mom to get her eyes examined because her worries were getting the best of her. We congratulated Joyce for taking a positive step in her diabetes care.

We explained to Joyce we would need to dilate and carefully look at the back of both eyes. We assured her that we would describe all the steps in the eye examination and explain their significance as well as our findings. She needed a dye test, or a fluorescein angiogram, to help us assess the retina circulation. With all the information gathered, we were able to show Joyce and her son the changes which had occurred in her retina from her diabetes. She had swelling in the macula of both eyes (macular edema) as well as new blood vessels growing on the surface of the retina of both eyes (proliferative retinopathy). We explained the need for laser treatment and were able to begin treatment that day. We gave Joyce and her son a booklet about diabetic retinopathy to read at home and encouraged them to return for follow-up visits with questions. We also spent time discussing diabetes and getting an understanding of some of the difficulties Joyce was having with diabetes management. Joyce's particular problem was with her weight, binge eating, and food choice.

We recommended that Joyce see a diabetes educator and a dietitian, who helped Joyce adjust her diet, learn about carbohydrate counting, and begin a walking program at a local mall. Joyce's vision has improved slightly over several months with better control of her sugar, and she is very glad we have been able to stabilize her vision.

Your ophthalmologist will likely have colored drawings and sketches in the office to explain his/her findings. Don't be afraid to ask him or her to explain unfamiliar words or describe your problem through a picture or an eye model. These visual aids will help you understand the diagnosis.

Eye Examinations

I don't like people messing with my eyes, but I'm afraid of going blind. How can I get up the nerve to have my eyes examined?

We hear this from many patients. It is very natural to fear the unknown. Sometimes it is helpful to bring a friend or family member to the examination with you. I have even had patients ask their pastors to come along with them. Patients tell me that enlisting a friend or family member as a driver helps them get up the nerve to follow through with examination appointments and tests. I make a habit of noting what goals my diabetic patients are pursuing, such as walking and weight loss. I try to encourage small goals at every visit.

What does the comprehensive diabetic eye examination consist of?

There are several steps to the comprehensive eye examination. These steps will be completed at the discretion of your ophthalmologist and in varying order, depending on the doctor's routine.

- ❖ symptoms: blurry vision, pain, floaters
- ❖ general medical history: medical and surgical history
- ❖ allergies to medications
- ❖ a list of your medications
- ❖ family history: especially for glaucoma or retinal problems
- ❖ social history: smoking, alcohol, drug use, employment status
- ❖ ocular history: any history of lazy eye (amblyopia), cross-eye (strabismus), injury to the eye, previous laser treatment or surgery, prior low vision evaluation
- ❖ checking of visual acuity with your glasses
- ❖ refraction (checks the prescription for the glasses)
- ❖ pupil assessment
- ❖ motility assessment (tests how the eye muscles work)
- ❖ visual field assessment (tests the side vision)
- ❖ Amsler grid
- ❖ slit lamp examination
- ❖ glaucoma test or intraocular pressure assessment
- ❖ dilated examination of the fundus

Which Eye Is Having a Problem?

Cover one eye and then the other. For example, if the visual problem is in your right eye, when you cover the right eye with your hand, the problem should disappear.

Symptoms

The most common complaint with any eye disease is *blurry vision*. This particular symptom is especially common for diabetics because of fluctuating sugars. The extra sugar in your body is converted into a substance called sorbitol. Sorbitol accumulates inside the lens of the eye. Sorbitol acts like a sponge and draws additional water into the lens. The lens changes shape and your refraction changes. It is like wearing someone else's glasses. This change is usually temporary.

Blurry vision can also result from swelling in the retina itself. The swelling usually occurs in the macula. You may notice that when you look straight ahead, the central area is blurry and the periphery or side vision is sharp. Macular edema needs evaluation to prevent further vision loss. It requires treatment.

Cataracts are common in diabetics and cause blurry and decreased vision. Diminished contrast, halos around lights, glare, and double vision which disappears when that eye is covered are also common. People may have more difficulty at distance or near depending on the type of cataract which has developed.

Foreign body sensation is a feeling like someone threw sand in your eyes. Many older patients develop dry eye syndrome accompanied by mild redness, intermittent blurry vision, and a gritty sensation in the eyes. Our tears are very complex and contain a liquid portion, a mucus portion, and an oily portion. If this mixture is unbalanced, we can develop a dry eye problem. I explain to patients that this is analogous to driving around with mud on your windshield and no windshield wiper fluid. We often prescribe artificial tears for dry eye syndrome, as well as warm compresses to the lids.

Pain is not a common symptom with diabetes. Sharp pain which is unrelenting is always an indication to see an eye doctor immediately even if you do not have diabetes. Usually eye pain is accompanied by tearing and sensitivity to light. Pain can be due to a corneal abrasion, or scratch of the cornea. Corneal abrasions tend to require more time to heal in diabetics.

Pain can also occur from infections of the cornea such as herpes infections. There are two types of herpes infections to which a diabetic may be susceptible, because the immune system is not as strong. Shingles, caused by herpes zoster, can attack the face and eye. Nongenital herpes, or type 1 herpes simplex, can also affect the lids and cornea.

Neovascular glaucoma is a type of glaucoma in which new blood vessels grow in the eye's drainage angle and plug it up. Because the eye is constantly making fluid, the new vessels make it impossible for the fluid to leave the eye. The pressure in the eye then skyrockets, and patients may complain of severe pain, headache, nausea, tearing, and photophobia. This type of glaucoma is more common in patients who have had untreated proliferative disease or a history of a central retinal vein occlusion (a plugged-up major vein in the retina).

Redness can occur for a variety of reasons: inflammation in the eye, infection, injury, allergy, elevated pressure in the eye, or bleeding under the conjunctiva. Redness may be accompanied by other symptoms such as pain and/or tearing. Redness accompanied by pain or vision loss should be evaluated immediately.

Bleeding under the conjunctiva is probably one of the most alarming conditions for patients but is generally not harmful. A large blood spot covers the white of the eye. This is called a subconjunctival hemorrhage. A small blood vessel in the conjunctiva, the clear covering over the sclera, has broken. This can occur from rubbing the eye, using blood thinners like aspirin or Coumadin, straining with coughing or constipation, high blood pressure, or contact lens wear. This blood spot can take several weeks to clear.

Itching can occur with dry eyes or blepharitis, inflammation of the eyelashes, or seasonal allergy. Cool compresses applied using a clean washcloth can often alleviate some of the desire to "scratch your eyes out."

Rapid onset of diplopia, or *double vision*, is cause for alarm in a diabetic and should be evaluated promptly. Usually our two eyes work together to look up and down, right and left. In double vision, the diabetes has caused the blood supply to the nerves to diminish; the nerve is demonstrating ischemia and is not working properly. There are specific nerves which stimulate specific muscles which move the eye. Any nerve can be affected and can cause one or more of the muscles not to work. The balance between the eyes is disturbed, and the patient sees double. Often the double vision will resolve over several weeks to months. However, any double vision accompanied by pain needs to be evaluated right away. Double vision with pain and a change of pupil size can be life threatening and should be taken seriously.

Reduced peripheral visual field can occur in patients with a history of diabetic retinopathy who have required extensive panretinal photocoagulation or laser treatments for their retinal disease. In patients with proliferative diabetic retinopathy, the laser has proven itself effective in preventing vision loss. It is an acceptable side effect to lose some peripheral vision in order to save your central, or reading vision. Other unacceptable causes of peripheral field loss include glaucoma and retinal detachment, which can occur in patients with diabetes.

Nyctalopia (nick-ta-lope-ee-a), or *difficulty with dark adaptation*, is not uncommon in patients with proliferative diabetic retinopathy who have undergone laser treatment. There are two types of photoreceptors, or electrical connectors within the retina. The rods assist with night and side vision and are located in the peripheral retina. The cones assist with color and reading vision and are located in the central macula. When panretinal photocoagulation (PRP) is performed, the laser spots are applied to the peripheral retina in order to promote the new blood vessels to disappear. As a consequence, the peripheral retina is lasered and some of the rods are destroyed. Thus, to save your sight, night vision becomes a little more difficult. This means that going from bright sunlight into a dark movie theater and vice versa will take more adaptation and more time than before you had laser surgery.

Floaters are opacities which float across one's visual field. Patients describe them as spider webs, blobs, and fine speckles. They move as you move your eye and can cause intermittent blurry vision. Floaters can be caused by bleeding inside the eye or by separation of the vitreous

CHRISTINE
"Do not allow insurance to restrict access to your ophthalmologist"

One Saturday while I was on call, Christine, a twenty-eight-year-old woman who had been diabetic for fifteen years, called me about some eye problems. She told me that she had been followed very closely at a clinic specializing in diabetes. However, over the last five years, she had not received an eye examination. She had no eye symptoms until today, when she noted some blurriness in her vision from her left eye. She called and wanted me to examine her.

Christine was a well-dressed, slim woman. She was accompanied by a supportive boyfriend. Her vision was not very good. With her glasses on, she could only see 20/40 from her right eye and 20/80 from her left. She probably would not have passed the vision requirement for driving had she been tested. When I dilated her eyes, I saw that she had severe retinopathy, high-risk proliferative diabetic retinopathy, and macular edema in both eyes. The growth of neo-vascularization was so severe that it was lifting the macula in her left eye. The macula, as you recall, is the most sensitive part of the retina.

Out of curiosity and concern, I asked her why she had stopped coming in for her eye examinations. She said she knew that annual eye examinations were important, but she had been laid off from her job for the last six months. She was currently working in a temporary position moving cargo at the airport, but this new job did not provide health coverage. She was hoping that she would find a permanent position soon with benefits. After hearing this story, I sadly realized that this attractive young woman would probably never regain her vision because she did not have insurance. I told her that I would go over with her what she needed, and that our practice and the hospital would make financial arrangements to help her out.

What Christine needed was laser treatment for her proliferative retinopathy, laser treatment for her macular edema, and surgery to release the scar tissue that was pulling on her macula. Ideally, the macular edema would be treated first, because laser treatment for proliferative retinopathy can make macular edema worse. However, we could not delay the laser treatment for her proliferative diabetic retinopathy because the eyes were quite severely damaged; we ended up treating both conditions at the same time.

Over a two-week period, Christine received three laser treatments to each eye. She then underwent surgery three weeks after I initally examined her. All in all, she had a satisfactory outcome. Her vision declined slightly following the laser surgery and the vitrectomy operation for the scar tissue in her left eye. However, after about eight weeks, her vision stabilized. Her vision was 20/50 in her right eye and 20/200 in the left.

However, I just couldn't help thinking what we could have done for her if she had come in earlier. Nobody can second-guess nature, but I predict we would have saved more of Christine's vision. She had assumed that she had to have insurance to see us and did not realize that special arrangements could be made. After Christine's experience, I now emphasize to every patient that vision is very important and that in diabetes, once vision is lost, you cannot regain it. I tell all my patients not to let insurance issues get in the way of medical care.

jelly from the retina, a posterior vitreous detachment (PVD) or, in diabetics, a combination of both.

Posterior vitreous detachments are a result of the natural aging process that occur in 70 percent of people by the time they reach age eighty. Posterior vitreous detachments can occur earlier in life in diabetics. The detached jelly can be very annoying without actually causing vision loss. Usually with time, the blob in your vision becomes less noticeable. Floaters associated with flashing lights need prompt attention, as this may represent an early tear in the retina.

A vitreous hemorrhage inside the eye can be very upsetting to any diabetic patient. Your vision can drop quickly to barely being able to see your hand or count fingers in front of your face. This can be very frightening. This sudden loss in vision often means that more bleeding from new blood vessels has occurred inside your eye. The new blood vessels grow along your retinal surface like ivy grows along a building face.

When this occurs, your ophthalmologist should examine you at a mutually convenient time to confirm the diagnosis. Your ophthalmologist will likely perform an ultrasound test to evaluate the health of the retina and to make sure that no retinal detachment has occurred. Just as the blood inside the eye blocks your view of the world, so your ophthalmologist's view of your retina is equally blocked. Your ophthalmologist may have you sleep on several pillows in an effort to use gravity to help the blood settle to the bottom of your eye.

Flashing lights, or photopsias, usually occur in both the dark and light; the flashing may not be continual. Often this signifies the pulling of the jelly on the retina. The retina is unable to distinguish this pulling from light shined on it and responds with a flashing light sensation. A migraine may also cause the sensation of flashing lights; however, these lights have a jagged, scintillating pattern across your visual field and are called visual aura.

General Medical History

Knowing how long you have had diabetes is very important. The longer the duration of diabetes, the more likely you will develop some form of retinopathy. Nephropathy or kidney problems, neuropathy or nerve problems, heart conditions, high blood pressure, high cholesterol, and foot problems are other complications related to diabetes. It is important that your ophthalmologist be up-to-date on your kidney function, blood pressure status, and cholesterol function. All these factors interrelate and can cause worsening of your macular edema.

A history of kidney stones is important, as some

glaucoma medications, such as acetazolamide, are best avoided if you have a history of stones.

Allergies

Medications such as sulfa drugs or iodine-based drugs are important. Sulfa drugs are used in a few of the oral and topical glaucoma medications. Indocyanine green (ICG) is a dye occasionally used to assess the choroidal circulation. Patients with allergies to shellfish and other iodine-containing substances, such as IUP dye, need to inform their ophthalmologist. Your health care provider may ask you to explain what type of reaction a particular drug causes; for example, hives or shortness of breath.

Medications

Asthma or emphysema is important as it can be exacerbated by some glaucoma medications called beta-blockers. Other medications like Glucophage (metformin) can cause renal failure when taken with iodinated dyes. While fluorescein is not an iodinated dye, indocyanine green (ICG) is an iodinated dye often used in ophthalmology to perform another dye test. Glucophage needs to be stopped seventy-two hours in advance of ICG testing and cannot be resumed until seventy-two hours after the test. Your doctor needs a list of your medications. For your own safety, you should always carry a list of your medications and allergies in the event of an emergency. Having this list laminated to carry in your wallet or purse is an excellent idea.

Family History

Glaucoma and retinal detachments can run in families. It is important that your doctor be aware of these conditions.

Social History

You might think that your social history is no one else's business. Your doctor and the staff must keep your medical history confidential. However, there are many things in your social history which can affect your eyes. Drinking and smoking in excess can affect the optic nerve. Eating raw meat can put you at risk for eye infections. Traveling to exotic countries can expose you to parasitic infections which can also affect the eye. Sexually transmitted diseases can affect the eye and cause infection and inflammation.

Knowing the type of job you do and what your visual demands are at work can help your ophthalmologist arrive at the best treatment option for you. A person who always works at the computer may require an intermediate prescription and be unhappy if the doctor doesn't automatically prescribe this type of lens. Knowing the distance you travel for treatment can help the doctor in planning laser sessions that are more convenient for you.

A job that involves significant air travel must be considered in planning ahead for surgery. Your surgeon may need to perform a procedure, for example, which removes the jelly in the eye and replaces this with an air or gas bubble. While that bubble is inside your eye, you may be unable to travel by air and you may need to adjust your work schedule.

If you are unemployed or don't have insurance, your doctor may be able to refer you to many of the special assistance programs for the needy which can help to provide medications and eyedrops (see Appendix D for an extensive list). He or she can suggest a social worker who is an expert in helping you get the assistance you may need to manage your diabetes.

The use of alcohol and cigarettes has been shown to elevate blood glucose levels. Cigarettes are also a risk factor for developing the wet type of macular degeneration, a separate cause of vision loss in adults over age fifty.

Past Ocular History

Your doctor wants to know the past history of your eyes. Have they ever been injured? Did you have a lazy eye, or amblyopia (am-blee-ope-ee-a), as a child? A lazy eye usually does not see as well and may have been associated with a weak muscle or cross-eye when you were young. If the physician is unaware that this eye has been lazy (it is not always apparent), he may initiate an expensive workup which includes CT scanning or other costly imaging tests. If you have had previous laser or retinal surgery, you will need to tell the ophthalmologist. This is especially important if the laser treatment is recent. It may take time to see improvement, and your doctor may want to delay additional therapy if he or she knows that you have had recent procedures. Only you as a patient can request your records. If you plan on seeing a new eye doctor, ask for your old records and bring them with you.

Visual Acuity

Visual acuity is a measurement of how well your eyes see standard letters at a given distance. Standard visual acuity is usually measured with Snellen letters, just like your weight is measured in pounds or your height is measured in inches. Snellen visual acuity ranges from 20/10 to 20/400. Most people refer to perfect vision as 20/20. Many individuals actually see better than this. The upper number is the standard test distance. For example, if a person has 20/200 visual acuity, this means that person can see at 20 feet (6 meters) what a normal person can see at 200 feet (60 meters).

Your visual acuity is assessed separately for each eye, usually with your glasses, to obtain the best possible visual acuity reading. After cataract surgery, before your glasses are changed, you may see better without your glasses. Your doctor will check your vision in such a manner that your best acuity is obtained. This measure will be recorded in your chart.

Refraction

This is the process by which your doctor checks you for glasses using a phoropter or single lens held in front of each eye. A phoropter looks like a giant pair of elephant-sized glasses with many knobs and dials. The doctor tests one eye at a time and asks you the monotonous question, "Which is better, 1 or 2?" Remember, this is not a test. Despite the fact that you can feel anxious at this point with flashbacks from grade school, there are no right or wrong answers, so relax. Refraction shows you two different pictures and lets you pick the better picture of the two. The ophthalmologist will adjust the phoropter settings every time you identify one picture as significantly better than the other. Eventually, you will see two pictures that look fairly similar and you will be unable to distinguish which is the better one. When you find it difficult to pick a better picture, tell your doctor that there isn't much of a difference. The ophthalmologist will prescribe these settings in the phoropter.

Most retina specialists do not perform refraction to dispense glasses. They will refract you only to determine your best visual potential for diagnostic purposes. They will most likely leave your glasses prescription in the hands of a general ophthalmologist or optometrist.

Pupil Assessment

Pupil reaction is examined to insure that the neural or electric part of your visual system is intact. When light falls on the retina, a nerve impulse travels from the retina to the optic nerve, then via a complex path through the brain; this is the afferent pathway, or pathway *to* the brain. The pathway *from* the brain is called the efferent pathway and returns an impulse from the brain to the pupils, causing them to constrict. The pupils constrict with bright light and dilate in darkness. Failure to react may indicate a diabetic neuropathy, a problem in the nerves from the brain or a problem in the pathway to the brain, specifically with the retina or optic nerve.

Motility Assessment

Misalignment of the eyes can occur from diabetes. Various nerves stimulate or innervate the muscles which move the eye. These nerves originate from the brain or cranial cavity and are therefore called cranial nerves. Cranial nerves III and VI may be affected by diabetes. With a III nerve palsy, the eyes are misaligned vertically and the affected eye appears turned down and out. The lid on that side may also be droopy. With a VI nerve palsy, the eyes are misaligned horizontally. The involved eye usually looks turned in and is unable to turn out.

Amsler Grid

An Amsler grid is a test of your central 10 degrees of vision (see Figure 3.2). This test is performed with each

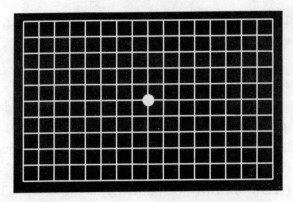

Figure 3.2 **Amsler grid**

eye separately. In older patients, glasses often have a portion of the lenses which give extra power for reading. This portion is called the bifocal. Sometimes, you can see the bifocal, which is demarcated by a horizontal line in the glasses. The part below the line is the bifocal. You will be asked to fixate on the dot in the center using your bifocal segment. Point out the areas where the lines are very wavy, missing, gray, or very blurry. This usually reflects a change in your macula and can be useful to your physician.

Slit Lamp Examination

This is performed with a lighted microscope and magnifies the front portion of your eye (see Figure 3.3). This machine has a chin rest in which you comfortably rest your chin while the doctor uses a slit-shaped beam of light to examine your eyes. The slit lamp allows the examination of the eyelids, cornea, anterior chamber, iris, and lens in magnified detail. Occasionally, very small blood vessels can grow on the surface of your iris. Often, they are most easily visualized at the pupil border. Neovascularization (new blood vessels) of the iris is often called rubeosis.

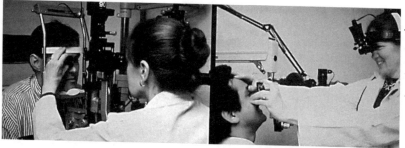

Figure 3.3 **Examination with slit lamp (left) and examination with indirect ophthalmoscope (right)**

Glaucoma Test

The eye pressure will be checked, usually with applanation. Some patients refer to this part of the examination as the glaucoma test. An anesthetic or numbing drop which contains fluorescein, a yellow-based vegetable dye, is instilled in each eye. A special flat tonometer attached to the slit lamp microscope is moved close to your eye until it gently touches the surface of the eye (the cornea); then the doctor will read your pressure off an attached pressure gauge. This test does not hurt. Most patients don't even notice that the doctor or technician took the pressure because it causes no pain and uses no bright light. The test takes only a second to perform. Some offices use a puff of air to check pressure, but most ophthalmologists use the applanation method because it is far more accurate.

Gonioscopy is a specialized examination that evaluates the drainage angle in the front of the eye with magnification using a special contact lens applied to the eye. It does not hurt at all, because the doctor uses a special anesthetic drop to numb the eye. People who routinely wear contact lenses don't need numbing drops to be able to tolerate their contact lenses. Your doctor simply wants to ensure your comfort. This part of the examination is only done if your doctor suspects narrow drainage angles, notices elevated eye pressure, suspects glaucoma, or sees new blood vessels growing on your iris. Once the examination is finished, the doctor will easily remove the contact lens.

Dilation

The slit lamp can also be used to examine the natural lens inside your eye as well as the back lining of your eye, the retina. Since your pupils are dilated, the entire retina can be carefully examined. Special handheld lenses in a range of powers are used by the ophthalmologist to evaluate the retina. These lenses do not touch your eye but focus bright light into your eye so that the retina can be magnified. Indirect ophthalmoscopy involves the use of a special head lamp that looks like a cross between a miner's hat and a virtual reality headset to look at the periphery of the retina. Once again, the eye specialist will use large lenses to image your retina. These lenses will be held several inches away from your eye. These lights are very bright and may temporarily bleach your vision. The doctor will give you a few minutes to recover. Your vision will return to normal following the examination.

What is a dye test, or fluorescein angiogram?

Diabetes causes damage to the retinal blood vessels and can result in closure of the vessels as well as leakage. In diabetes, the blood vessels can close off and prevent blood from flowing to vital areas of the retina. It is as though someone stepped on one of your garden hoses so patches of your lawn are yellow rather than green. In other places, the capillaries, or smallest blood vessels in the retina may develop outpouches or microaneurysms. At these points, leakage may occur, which causes swelling of the surrounding retina. The leakage is very similar to a garden hose with many holes in it that causes water to drip all over your sidewalk.

The dye test helps determine where the leaks sprang from (see Figure 3.4). The dye test can also detect areas of ischemia or nonperfusion. Ischemia indicates areas of the retina which don't get enough blood supply.

The dye is vegetable based and contains no iodine. It is injected into a vein using a small butterfly needle. The injection lasts ten seconds or less. One in fifty people may feel a little nauseous as the dye is being injected or shortly afterward. The dye is a bright yellow and will leave your skin and urine dark yellow for about twenty-four hours. The majority of patients have no side effects from this test.

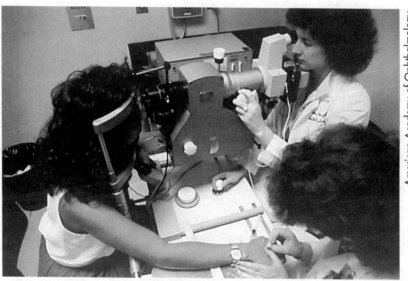

American Academy of Ophthalmology

Figure 3.4 **Patient undergoing fluorescein angiography**

The test requires the use of a camera and film. The film is developed in about one to two hours. Usually, the patient is allowed to return home after the test; the doctor will make an appointment to discuss the results with you. Many offices now no longer use film but utilize a computer to store images previously captured on film. Digital imaging is being used much more frequently; in this case, the pictures of the dye in the retinal blood vessels are immediately available. Your doctor may either schedule you for laser treatment or begin it immediately.

When is ultrasonography used for diabetic retinopathy?

Ultrasonography is used for diabetic retinopathy evaluations whenever the view of the back of the eye, the retina, is obscured by either a dense cataract or blood inside the eye. The ultrasound used to evaluate the retina is similar to that used to check fetuses by obstetricians. High frequency waves delivered through a special probe bounce sound off the eye and give various echoes, which create a black and white image of the inside of the eye. Ultrasonography is used most frequently to "see through" blood inside the eye which obscures an ophthalmologist's ability to visualize the retina clearly. It ensures that the retina is not detached.

What should I bring with me to my eye examination?

It is common for a patient to show up for an eye examination without his or her glasses or list of medications. Patients may be upset about their old glasses yet forget to bring them along. They may be upset about a new medication which causes side effects but forget the name of the medication. They may be out of their eyedrops and not know the name. They may come to a new doctor for a second opinion but not bring along their old records.

You need to request your records from your previous physician. A copy of your last fluorescein angiogram or dye test might save you the expense of another such test. (Remember, only you can give permission for your records to be transferred.)

Even if you are seeking a second opinion, your eyes will probably be dilated again. Bring your sunglasses with you to the examination.

Doctors do want to help you; unfortunately, they do not have ESP and cannot read your mind. The prepared patient often seems to be the patient who wants to get better. Doctors may not admit this, but it is much easier to provide care for someone who takes responsibility for his or her own health care.

To sum up, remember to bring old records (including a fluorescein angiogram), a list of medications, your glasses (whether you like them or not), and a pair of sunglasses.

What might the ophthalmologist or eye care specialist see inside my eye?

Diabetic retinopathy is often separated into two types: nonproliferative or proliferative. Proliferate means to grow and multiply. As discussed earlier, proliferative disease in diabetic retinopathy means that new blood vessels are growing along the surface of the retina, like ivy grows along the side of a brick building. Nonproliferative disease indicates that there are changes in the retina; however, there is no sign of new blood vessels growing on the surface. Background diabetic retinopathy (BDR or NPDR) is usually evaluated yearly, unless there is accompanying macular edema which may require either laser treatment or observation. Occasionally, your two eyes may be asymmetric or at different stages and your doctor may wish to see you sooner. If you have other eye conditions such as glaucoma, cataracts, or macular degeneration, you may also need to be seen more frequently.

If you are planning a pregnancy, you should be evaluated before you are actually pregnant. A number of hormone changes take place during pregnancy and the body requires a lot of energy to grow a healthy baby. The pregnant woman with preexisting diabetes is at risk for increased difficulty in controlling her sugars. Studies have shown that pregnancy can increase the risk of diabetic retinopathy progressing. The risk of progression can vary between 10 and 55 percent, depending on the baseline degree of retinopathy prior to pregnancy.

Besides the initial level of retinopathy, the glycosolated hemoglobin level (Hemoglobin A_{1c}) and how long you've had diabetes are other risk factors associated with the progression of retinopathy. The degree of improvement in diabetes control through the fourteenth week of pregnancy also is associated with progression of retinopathy. For women with diabetic retinopathy contemplating pregnancy, strict control is recommended prior to becoming pregnant. Also, ensuring that your diabetic retinopathy has been evaluated prior to pregnancy and treated if necessary is equally important (see Chapter 9). The frequency of eye examinations depends on the initial findings of the ophthalmologist or eye care specialist. Women who develop gestational diabetes are not at increased risk for diabetic retinopathy and do not require close ophthalmology supervision during pregnancy.

How often should I have an eye examination?

Table 3.1 lists guidelines recommended by the American Academy of Ophthalmology and are published as part of the educational program, Diabetes 2000, which is a coordinated nationwide effort of many ophthalmologists and retina specialists to educate the public about preventive visual loss from diabetic retinopathy. A frequency schedule for evaluation is based on the first examination findings.

It should be emphasized that these guidelines apply to one eye. Your doctor may elect to see you more often if you also need to have your other eye treated or monitored.

How many spots of laser should I expect to receive?

Different kinds of laser are used to treat diabetic problems. Macular edema is treated differently than proliferative diabetic retinopathy. The number of spots each patient receives is always different. The spot size placed can vary as can your response to the laser. Some people may require less laser to induce regression of the proliferative disease. Another person may have poorly controlled blood pressure making it difficult to treat the macular edema with just one treatment.

Not everyone I know with diabetes sees an eye doctor. Are there some diabetics who don't need an eye examination?

No. It has been clearly demonstrated that diabetes takes time to cause damage to the eye. One study showed that

Table 3.1 MANAGEMENT GUIDELINES

Diabetic status of retina	Follow-up (months)	Laser	Fluorescein angiography	Color fundus photography
Normal to minimal	12	No	No	No
Nonproliferative DR without macular edema	6–12	No	No	Rarely
Nonproliferative DR with macular edema, not clinically significant	4–6	No	Occasionally	Occasionally
Nonproliferative DR with clinically significant macular edema	3–4	Yes	Yes	Yes
Preproliferative DR	3–4	Occasionally	Occasionally	Occasionally
Non–high-risk proliferative DR	2–3	Occasionally	Occasionally	Occasionally
Non–high-risk proliferative DR with clinically significant macular edema	2–3	Occasionally	Yes	Yes
High-risk proliferative DR	3–4	Yes	Occasionally	Yes
High-risk proliferative DR not amenable to laser	1–6	Occasionally	No	If possible

after nine years of diabetes, retinopathy had developed in 50 percent of the study patients; after twenty years, 100 percent had retinopathy. Prevention is one very important aspect of diabetic care. Unfortunately, a 1989 study noted that only 49 percent of adults diagnosed with diabetes received a *dilated* eye examination.

Diabetes is the leading cause of new blindness in the United States. Despite the advances and available treatments of retinopathy by laser and surgery, education of the public and health care professionals has lagged in emphasizing the importance of a dilated eye examination by a trained ophthalmologist or retinal specialist.

Do I need to have my eyes dilated?

Yes. All diabetics need a dilated eye examination. A fully dilated pupil is necessary to ensure maximum visualization of the retina. In two studies, only 50 percent of diabetic eyes were correctly classified as to the presence and severity of the retinopathy if the pupils were not dilated. While no one likes the side effects of dilating drops—burning, blurry near vision, and light sensitivity—no one should put themselves at risk for preventable blindness.

In the future, devices called nonmydriatic cameras may be available to screen patients effectively without dilation of the eyes. These cameras are being developed as screening devices; however, the cameras do not check visual acuity or intraocular pressures (part of glaucoma screening). They just check for diabetic retinopathy.

My friend went blind from diabetes after she had her laser treatment and surgery. I am afraid to have my eyes examined because I might also go blind. Does laser treatment cause blindness?

This is perhaps the most common misperception about laser treatments. Many patients have the false belief that the laser causes blindness rather than preventing further loss of vision.

I explain to patients that diabetic retinopathy is best compared to a dam which has held back the water in a reservoir for years. Just as diabetic retinopathy takes years to develop, so the dam with its thick walls and hardy construction takes years to develop a tiny leak from the weathering of the elements. The ophthalmologist steps in to plug the ever-growing leaks and new blood vessels for a patient that hasn't received careful follow-up and treatment of his or her diabetes, cholesterol and blood pressure, just as the construction worker steps in to try and fix the leaking dam with its raging waters. The dam may burst just as the construction worker is trying to plug the leak. The unattended patient's vision drops precipitously just as the retina specialist or ophthalmologist starts using lots of laser. The patient associates his or her decline in vision with the laser treatments, rather than the long-standing diabetes and medical problems. In many cases, routine dilated eye examinations by an ophthalmologist, retinal specialist, or optometrist trained in retina care may have prevented the severe vision loss in the patient.

Diabetes is a disease that is always with our patients. There are good days and bad days. A patient with diabetes lives in a world filled with do's and don'ts. It is much too easy to have one's psychological well-being fluctuate with a "good sugar" or a "bad sugar." The more you learn about diabetes and how it affects the eyes, the more you will understand that many of the complications of diabetes are preventable. Prevention can only take place with knowledge and communication. Your eye doctor wants you to ask questions. Knowledge is power. Don't let your diabetes control you—learn to control your diabetes.

4

Medicines for Diabetic Retinopathy

Any patient would much prefer to take a pill or an eye-drop rather than undergo surgery. It's easy to take a pill at home, without interruption of daily routine. And a pill appears to be safer. With surgery, there are risks of anesthesia and risks of the surgery itself.

There are some very effective medications for the treatment of diabetes, especially Type II, or non-insulin dependent diabetes. However, at present, no medication seems effective for treating diabetic retinopathy.

Medications

Insulin

Prior to Dr. Frederick Banting's discovery of insulin earlier this century, Type I diabetes was a uniformly fatal disease. The injection of insulin along with adjustment of lifestyle, including diet and exercise, has vastly increased the life span of today's patients with diabetes. However, chronic complications now develop from the many years of high blood glucose levels. One of these complications is diabetic retinopathy.

About ten to twenty years ago, there was a debate as to whether insulin caused diabetic retinopathy. We now know that insulin, especially the highly purified insulin made from bioengineering (such as Humulin, Novolin) does not lead to worsening of retinopathy. In fact, good glucose control from multiple injections of insulin a day in patients with Type I diabetes can prevent the development of diabetic retinopathy and slow down its progression. These findings were shown in the Diabetes Control and Complications Trial (DCCT).

The use of insulin for Type II diabetes is more controversial. Insulin injection can lead to weight gain, which then can increase the risk of strokes and heart attacks in older patients with diabetes. This is not to say that good glucose control is not necessary for Type II diabetics. Good glucose control is important, but a better method may be diet, exercise, and weight loss rather than multiple injections of insulin. However, there is no evidence to suggest that insulin is harmful to the eyes and patients should use insulin if it is prescribed to control their blood sugar.

Oral Antidiabetic Agents

After diet, weight loss, and exercise, patients with Type II diabetes may be prescribed an oral antidiabetic agent (see Table 4.1). Basically, these agents work by stimulating the insulin receptor. In Type II diabetes, these oral agents can be very effective. Over time, however, certain patients

Table 4.1   ORAL ANTIDIABETIC AGENTS

Class	Name of Drug	Manufacturer
Biguanides	Glucophage	Bristol-Myers-Squibb
Glucosidase inhibitors	Precose	Bayer Pharmaceuticals
Sulfonylureas	Amaryl	Hoechst Marion Roussel
	Diabeta	Hoechst Marion Roussel
	Diabenese	Pfizer
	Glucotrol	Pfizer
	Glucotrol XL	Pfizer
	Glynase	Pharmacia & Upjohn
	Micronase	Pharmacia & Upjohn

with Type II diabetes will need insulin to help control blood sugar.

Oral agents, through their ability to keep blood glucose levels normal, are beneficial to the eyes. However, they do not directly have any effect on retinopathy.

Aspirin

As we discuss in Chapter 6, diabetic retinopathy occurs in part because there is closure of the small blood vessels in the retina. One theory is that the blood clots off in the blood vessels, causing blood flow to slow or stop. Using this thinking, a number of studies have involved drugs that "thin out" the blood to determine whether the closure of blood vessels might be prevented as well as the progression of diabetic retinopathy. One of the drugs studied was aspirin.

SUZANNE
"Stay away from fast food"

Suzanne is a fifty-eight-year-old woman who presented to my office after noticing some changes in her
vision. At the time I saw her, she had had diabetes for
twenty years. She was taking pills to control her diabetes, but her diabetes doctor had discussed the need
to start insulin.

She was slightly overweight. Her vision was 20/30
in the right eye and 20/100 in the left. She was having
problems doing fine tasks such as reading. Because she
worked with documents at her job, she was finding it
increasingly difficult to work. After dilating her pupils, I
examined the retinas of both eyes. On the right, she
had early proliferative diabetic retinopathy with macular edema. On the left, she had proliferative diabetic
retinopathy, vitreous hemorrhage, and macular edema.

What Suzanne required was laser treatment to
both her eyes for both the proliferative diabetic
retinopathy and the macular edema. Although she was
reluctant to have laser treatment at first, she under-
stood and agreed to it. Suzanne also wanted to know
about the risks of insulin on the eyes, because her
endocrinologist was thinking of prescribing insulin to
treat her diabetes.

Insulin can be a very effective drug to control
blood sugar when it is needed. I told her insulin by
itself does not damage the eyes, but there are risks
of using it. Studies have shown that good glycemic

control helps retard the progression of diabetic eye disease. However, most of the studies were done in younger diabetics. I told her what I tell all my older patients with diabetes. I recommend that they combine a program of diet control, weight loss, and exercise. If they can adhere to this regimen, they will often not need insulin.

After seeing her on several visits, I found out that Suzanne did very little exercise and ate fast foods often. I again emphasized to her the importance of a diet containing fruits and vegetables, weight loss, and exercise. After several more visits, she reported that she was able to adopt the exercise regimen without much difficulty. However, she was having trouble staying off the fast-food diet and losing weight. I tried to figure out how to help her and one day, the solution became clear. The answer was apparent when she came to one of her appointments with her husband, Peter. He was also overweight. We discussed my suggestions for Suzanne's diet and it turned out that she was making a good effort. But with Peter's frequent requests for fast foods, Suzanne fell off her diet. After I discussed the need for good diet control, her husband agreed to be an active participant. On her subsequent visits, Suzanne reported good progress with diet control and weight loss. In fact, she lost so much weight that insulin did not need to be started.

Her eyes stabilized after the laser treatment. The vision in her left eye even improved a little, as the vitreous hemorrhage cleared.

In the Early Treatment Diabetic Retinopathy Study, approximately 3,711 patients with diabetic retinopathy were randomly assigned to receive either aspirin therapy or placebo for an average of five years. At the end of the study, there was no difference in the course of the diabetic retinopathy between the two groups. Patients treated with aspirin did not have a slower rate of progression. However, patients on aspirin also did not have a faster progression rate. Basically, the study showed that aspirin has no effect on diabetic retinopathy.

In addition to finding that aspirin had no effect on retinopathy, the ETDRS also found that aspirin had no effect on the severity or duration of vitreous hemorrhages. These results tell us that patients who are taking aspirin for their hearts, or to prevent strokes, do not need to stop their aspirin treatment. Aspirin taken for other reasons will not harm the eyes. In patients who have a vitreous hemorrhage, there is no compelling reason to stop taking aspirin. Some patients fear that aspirin will prolong or increase the blood in their eyes, but there in no evidence that aspirin treatment will cause these problems.

Experimental Drugs

Sorbinil

Laboratory experiments have shown that polyol can cause sugar-induced cataracts. Polyol is a substance that comes from the enzyme, aldose reductase. Experimental studies have shown that inhibitors of aldose reductase can reduce the formation of these cataracts. There are also suggestions that these inhibitors might also be effective in preventing diabetic retinopathy. Unfortunately, the only large clinical trial to date, the Sorbinil Retinopathy Trial, failed to show a beneficial effect. In addition, a proportion of patients had side effects from this medication and had to stop taking it.

The fact that the trial did not show an effect may not mean that aldose reductase inhibitors are not effective. First, this clinical trial studied only one inhibitor. There are quite a few others. Some may have fewer side effects and may be stronger aldose reductase inhibitors. Table 4.2 lists aldose reductase inhibitors that have been tested in humans. Second, the study may have been conducted for too short a period of time. We know from the Diabetes Control and Complications Trial that patients in prevention studies must be followed for a long time. The preventive effect may not be observed until three years after starting the therapy. In summary, scientists are still wondering whether this class of drugs might be effective.

ACE Inhibitors

There is some evidence that kidney failure affects the course of diabetic retinopathy. Recently, clinical trials have shown that one class of anti-high blood pressure medications can prevent kidney failure. This class of medications is called angiotensin converting enzyme inhibitors, ACE inhibitors for short. This class of drug is thought to protect against retinopathy in the following ways. ACE inhibitors can prevent kidney damage and prevent the buildup of toxins that might be bad for the blood vessels of the retina. Second, ACE inhibitors reduce blood pressure and may prevent damage to retinal blood vessels. Whether this class of drugs might be helpful is as yet unknown. Dr. Fong is

Table 4.2   ALDOSE REDUCTASE INHIBITORS

Name	Developer
Alrestin	Ayerst, USA
Isodibut	Inst. Endocrin. Metab. Kiev, Russia
Ponsirestat	ICI, England
FK 366	Fujisawa, Japan
Tolrestat	Wyeth-Ayerst, USA
Epirestat	Ono, Japan
AD 5467	Takeda, Japan
Sorbinil	Pfizer, USA
Methosorbinil	Elsai, Japan
SNK 860	Sanwa, Japan
Alconil	Alcon, USA

conducting a study to determine whether this class of blood pressure medications is effective.

Eyedrops

There is no medication that can prevent the damage to the eyes that occurs from high sugar levels. However, eyedrops are used in the examination process, for treating glaucoma, and after surgery.

As part of your examination, eyedrops are routinely instilled to check the pressure inside your eye (see Figure 4.1). The eyedrops contain a yellow vegetable dye (fluorescein) and a topical anesthetic to numb the front of the eyes. The yellow dye can stain fabric, so don't let the drops drip onto your clothing! The anesthetic drop is necessary because it permits the tonometer, the instrument which checks pressure, to touch the front surface of the eye with maximum comfort. This is the most accurate way to check the pressure. The anesthetic allows the instrument to come close without causing you to blink. Because the anesthetic numbs your eye, you should remember to blink frequently for thirty minutes after your pressure has been checked.

The second set of eyedrops is used to enlarge the pupils for examination. As discussed in Chapter 3, dilated pupils

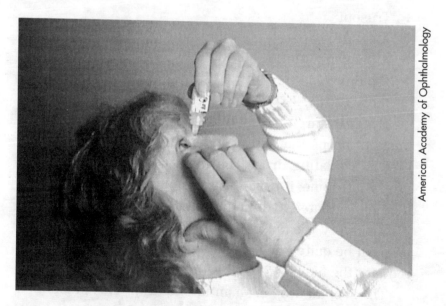

American Academy of Ophthalmology

*Figure 4.1 **The proper way of instilling eye drops: Tilt head back and use one hand to hold lower eyelid and the other to instill drops.***

allow examination of the lens, vitreous body, retina, and optic nerve. The dilating drops used in the examination last about six hours. During this time, you will be very sensitive to light, because the pupil will not be able to close down. In addition, if you don't need reading glasses, these eye-drops will make it difficult for you to see up close.

Eyedrops are also frequently used to treat glaucoma. As you recall, glaucoma is an eye disease where high pressures in the eye cause damage to the optic nerve, resulting in loss of vision. Eyedrops used for glaucoma reduce the pressure inside the eye. Common eyedrops used to treat glaucoma include:

❖ Betoptic®
❖ Pilocarpine®
❖ Timoptic®
❖ Propine®
❖ Trusopt®
❖ Xalatan®
❖ Alphagan®
❖ Iopidine®

Eyedrops are also used after surgery. There are three kinds of drops that are routinely used after surgery. The first is a dilating drop. The most commonly prescribed drop is atropine; it usually has a red cap. This drop keeps the pupils dilated and the muscles inside the eyes at rest. After surgery, the muscles in the eyes may "cramp up" and this can be quite uncomfortable. Using this atropine drop reduces the likelihood of this discomfort.

The second drop is an antibiotic drop. This prescribed drop is given to prevent an infection from developing. Eyes that have been operated on are at higher risk of infection. An antibiotic is usually instilled several times a day for a few weeks after the surgery.

The third drop is a steroid drop. Steroids reduce inflammation and help the healing process. The steroid used in eyedrops is not the kind that builds muscles. In fact, no muscles will be enhanced with this eyedrop. The main effect is to reduce discomfort and enhance healing.

Alternative Medicine

There is a great deal of interest in alternative treatments for diabetes and diabetic eye disease. Some of the ideas are quite interesting and may have merit. However, these ideas, without exception, have not been tested using modern scientific methods. Nevertheless, you may have heard of some of these treatments.

In traditional Chinese medicine (TCM), diabetes mellitus is thought to occur through an imbalance of the yin and yang, and the disorder of Zang-Fu (viscera). Diabetes mellitus develops because of excess "pulmonic heat," "stomach heat," and insufficiency of the kidney. Excessive heat of lung and stomach then consumes the body fluid and results in deficiency of "yin." The principle of treatment, therefore, is reducing heat, nourishing the "yin," and strengthening the kidney. Common prescriptions are composed of herbs such as *Radix trichosanthis*, *Rhizoma polygonati odorati*, *Radix scrophulariae*, raw *Gypsum fibrosum*, raw *Radix rehmanniae*, and *Radix glehniae*. *Flos buddlejae* and *Semen celosiae* may be helpful in patients with retinopathy. Although TCM practitioners prescribe these herbs, the mechanism of action for the ingredients has not been well documented and the treatments have not been studied with clinical trials.

Gymnema sylvestre is an extract of ayurvedic herbs used widely in traditional Eastern medication practice. The active ingredient in *Gymnema sylvestre* is "gymnemic acid" which prevents the taste buds from being activated by sugar molecules and keeps the intestine from absorbing sugar molecules. *Gymnema sylvestre* allegedly works by reducing the appetite for sweet-tasting food and by reducing the metabolic effects of sugar by lessening its absorption in the intestines.

The absence of an effective medication in Western medicine leads many patients with retinopathy to consider alternatives. However, there is little evidence that the alternatives are effective or even safe.

Summary

The best medicine to prevent diabetic retinopathy is good control of blood glucose levels. There are no medications that have been shown to specifically work on preventing retinopathy and vision loss. Alternative medicines may be helpful, but your choice of alternatives should be based on effectiveness and safety. Remember, good blood glucose control will reduce the chance of developing any retinopathy and lessen the chance of its progression.

5

Surgery for Diabetic Retinopathy

The first effective treatment for diabetic retinopathy was laser photocoagulation; it was first shown effective in the late 1960s. Since that time, numerous studies, including three from the National Institutes of Health (NIH)—the Diabetic Retinopathy Study, DRS; the Early Treatment Diabetic Retinopathy Study, ETDRS; and the Diabetic Retinopathy Vitrectomy Study, DRVS—have demonstrated that timely laser treatment and vitrectomy surgery when necessary can prevent blindness.

Treatment of Macular Edema

Laser treatment is very effective for treating macular edema. Diabetic macular edema can be present at any level of retinopathy. It causes dysfunction of the macula in the following ways: collection of fluid in the macula, decreased blood flow to the macula, wrinkling of the normally very smooth surface of the macula, and/or retinal hole formation. Ophthalmologists refer to macular edema as clinically significant or not. Clinically significant macular edema can be diagnosed when there is swelling near to or in the center of the retina. To determine whether the macular edema needs to be treated, ophthalmologists evaluate the macula through dilated pupils. If clinically significant macular edema is present, the ophthalmologist may choose to get some pictures of the retina (fundus photographs) and to perform fluorescein angiography (see Figure 5.1). Fluorescein angiography is done to pinpoint where the blood vessels are leaking. If the leaky areas are thought to be treatable, the ophthalmologist will likely perform laser surgery. The kind of laser treatment used for macular edema is called focal laser photocoagulation. Occasionally, the fluid is not focally located but diffusely leaking. The kind of laser treatment used for diffuse macular edema is called grid laser photocoagulation.

American Academy of Ophthalmology

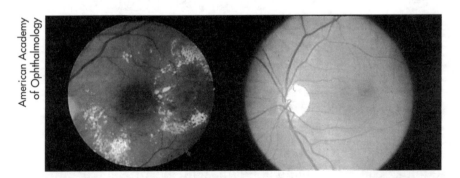

Figure 5.1 **Picture of the macula region of an eye without diabetic retinopathy (left); picture of the diabetic macular edema (right)**

When will the treatment start?

At your regular eye checkups, your eye doctor monitors the status of your retinas. One of the things that he or she looks for is the development of macular edema. If there is significant macular edema, your doctor will recommend a fluorescein angiography test to study it. If he or she feels that the edema needs to be treated, focal or grid laser treatment will be recommended. In most circumstances, you can take a few days to a few weeks to consider the treatment. Because many doctors like to have an updated angiogram when treating, you may need to undergo fluorescein angiography again if you delayed your decision to have the laser surgery performed.

What is the procedure like?

The focal laser surgery is done with the slit lamp (see Figure 5.2). The slit lamp is the instrument used to examine your eyes. You place your head on the slit lamp chin rest just as you would if you were being examined. After a numbing drop is instilled, a contact lens is placed on the eye to be treated. The contact lens is used to stabilize the eye and to deliver the laser beam.

When the surgery is performed, you will hear some clicks and see some bright lights. These are signs that the laser is making burns to seal up the leaky areas inside your eyes. The laser burns are made close to the very center of your vision. Multiple burns are often placed about one-tenth of a millimeter apart and about half a millimeter from the center of your vision (fovea). The fovea is usually avoided, because a burn placed there would lead to

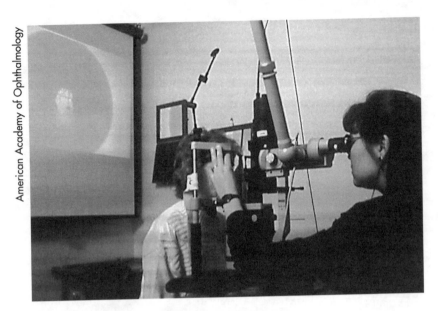

American Academy of Ophthalmology

Figure 5.2 **Patient receiving laser treatment**

instantaneous loss of vision. To avoid a foveal burn, your eye doctor will ask you to hold your head and eyes very still. The whole operation takes between ten and twenty minutes. Try not to look directly at the laser beam. If you are unsure, ask your doctor where you should look during the procedure.

Because the retina does not have touch or pain nerve fibers, no anesthesia is necessary. Usually, a drop of a numbing medication is used so that you will not feel the contact lens resting on your eye.

What are the benefits of the treatment and how successful is it?

Focal laser surgery is quite effective. A landmark study, the Early Treatment Diabetic Retinopathy Study, showed that eyes with macular edema treated with focal laser were 50 percent less likely to lose vision. However, the focal laser does not repair already damaged vision. *This is an important point.* The focal laser can prevent visual loss, but it cannot restore vision already lost.

The patient often questions the need for laser surgery when she or he can see perfectly well. Many patients think that laser surgery should be performed when their vision is bad. The exact opposite is true. Ideally, focal laser surgery should take place *before* any vision is lost. From the patient's perspective, however, this may be difficult to understand when nothing appears to be wrong. Remember, when focal laser surgery is performed on an eye with good vision, it is to prevent visual loss. You can ask your ophthalmologist to show you the leaky areas on your fluorescein angiogram. This will reassure you, when your vision is excellent, that preventive treatment is needed.

What are the risks of focal laser surgery?

As discussed, multiple burns are often placed about one-tenth of a millimeter apart and about half a millimeter from the center of your vision (fovea). The fovea has to be avoided because a burn placed there would lead to instantaneous and permanent loss of vision. While focal laser surgery is delicate, it is usually performed by experienced surgeons; therefore, an inadvertent burn in the fovea is quite uncommon.

Sometimes vision may temporarily decline after laser treatment. If you experience loss of vision, you should keep the following in mind: First, the treatment uses a bright light during the procedure. This bright light tends to bleach the

MARY
"Concerned about the laser"

Mary is a seventy-eight-year-old woman who was a trustee at one of the universities with which I was affiliated. The college president called to ask me to personally examine her, so my office scheduled an appointment for Mary for the following week. However, it was not until three reschedules later that she finally presented herself in my office.

Mary apologized for rescheduling her appointments and proceeded to tell me that she thought that her last ophthalmologist had treated her with the laser, but that it had caused some bleeding in her eyes. She was hesitant about coming in for her appointment because she was afraid of losing more vision from the treatment. She had been diabetic for twenty years and was taking both oral medications and insulin.

On my examination, Mary's vision was 20/25 in the right eye and 20/40 in the left. Pressure in the eyes was normal. After dilation of her pupils, I examined her retinas. In her right eye, there was extensive neovascularization. The left eye showed vitreous hemorrhage, neovascularization, and scars from previous laser treatment.

I told her that she had significant damage to the inside of her eyes. I explained to her the importance of keeping her eye appointments and the need for more laser treatment. After hearing my discussion about the effectiveness of laser surgery, she asked whether the laser might have caused the bleeding in her eyes. I told her that eyes with neovascularization (which she had) would tend to get worse over time. If no treatment was applied, the neovascularization would likely bleed and scar, pull on the retina, and cause visual loss. I told her that properly applied laser does not cause bleeding, and it looked like her previous treatment had been properly applied. I said that if she did not have additional laser surgery, she would likely lose more vision. Laser cannot cure diabetic retinopathy, and cannot always stop visual loss. Even if more laser was applied to both eyes, there was still a high chance of additional bleeding. However, if we were to stop treatment, she would likely continue to lose vision. Mary thought about it for a few more days and scheduled an appointment for the laser surgery.

My advice to her and to many of my patients is not to be overly worried about the harmful effects of the laser. Laser treatment overall does more good than harm. In eyes with severe neovascularization or in eyes with vitreous hemorrhage, laser treatment should not be delayed.

eyes immediately after surgery. Over the next half day or so, the vision will return. Second, if you notice little tiny dark spots in your vision, you are seeing the burns placed during the surgery. Most of the time, you will notice these dark spots less over the next several weeks. Third, if after several weeks, your vision is not as good as it was before the surgery, you may want to ask your eye doctor to examine you again. While it is possible for the focal laser surgery to cause worsening of vision, it is more likely that the disease process (the macular edema) has worsened your visual loss. You should remember that vision loss from macular edema does occur and this is the reason why focal laser surgery was recommended in the first place. Although neither you nor your doctor will ever know for sure, you may have lost more vision had the laser not been performed. Table 5.1 lists the risk of focal laser surgery.

Are there foods, drugs, or activities that I should avoid after focal laser surgery?

You should continue your diabetic diet and your medications. You can continue to take all medications before and after laser surgery. Surgical care following focal laser surgery is quite simple. No patch is usually applied and no drops are necessary. The patient can usually resume his or her normal activities as soon as the dilating drop wears off. However, because surgery is stressful, most patients do take the rest of the day off after the procedure.

Are other treatments available?

Sometimes, if the macular edema is very extensive, major surgery in the operating room is recommended. At present, there is no drug, eyedrop, or medication to treat macular edema. Maximizing blood pressure control, reducing elevated blood cholesterol, and improving kidney function have been shown to improve macular edema.

A small percentage of cases of macular edema will improve over time. Observation in this case is a viable

Table 5.1   POTENTIAL COMPLICATIONS OF SURGERY

Complications of Laser Surgery

Failure to achieve intent of surgery
Loss of central or side vision
Bleeding in eye
Early or late increase in pressure in eye (glaucoma)
Corneal burns
Damage to lens (cataract)
Retinal hole
Collection of fluid in back of eye
Damage to optic nerve
Damage to iris
Damage to intraocular lens implant, if present
Loss of vision or loss of eye

Complications of Anesthesia Injections Around the Eye

Perforation of eyeball
Destruction of optic nerve
Interference with circulation of retina
Possible drooping of eyelid
Respiratory depression
Hypotension (low blood pressure)
Loss of life
Stroke
Bleeding behind the eye

Complications of Vitrectomy Surgery

Failure to accomplish intent of surgery
Retinal detachment that may require additional surgery or may
    be inoperable
Vitreous hemorrhage
Infection
Elevated eye pressure (glaucoma)

continued

Table 5.1 *continued*

Complications of Vitrectomy Surgery *continued*

Poor healing or nonhealing corneal defects
Corneal clouding and scarring
Cataracts, which might require eventual or immediate removal of lens
Double vision
Eyelid droop
Loss of circulation to vital tissues in the eye, resulting in decrease or loss
    of vision
Permanent blindness
Loss of eye
Phthisis (disfigurement and shrinkage of eyeball)
Optic nerve injury
Closure of the eye's artery or vein

Complications of Retinal Surgery

Failure to accomplish intent of surgery
Retinal detachments that require additional surgery or may be inoperable
Vitreous hemorrhage
Hemorrhage under the retina
Change in eyeglass prescription
Infection
Elevated eye pressure (glaucoma)
Poor healing or nonhealing corneal defects
Corneal clouding and scarring
Cataracts, which might require eventual or immediate removal of lens
Double vision
Eyelid droop
Loss of circulation to vital tissues in the eye, resulting in decrease or loss
    of vision
Permanent blindness
Loss of eye
Phthisis (disfigurement and shrinkage of eyeball)

alternative. However, for clinically significant macular edema (CSME), research studies have shown that treatment is necessary to prevent the situation from worsening.

Treatment of Proliferative Diabetic Retinopathy

Neovascularization (growth of new blood vessels) can damage the eyes in several ways. First, the new blood vessels can bleed and lead to the buildup of blood within the eyes. This collection of blood obscures vision and leads to visual loss (see Figure 5.3). Another problem is that the new blood vessels can become scar tissue. In the process of maturing into a scar, the new blood vessels often contract and pull the retina off. A detached retina cannot function well and

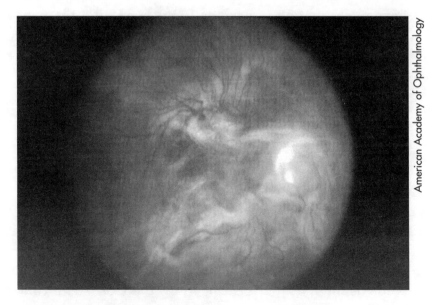

Figure 5.3 **Picture of proliferative diabetic retinopathy**

leads to further visual loss. When neovascularization is present, the eye is said to have proliferative diabetic retinopathy (PDR).

The best way to prevent these complications of neovascularization is early treatment. Laser treatment of retinal neovascularization is very effective and is called either scatter laser photocoagulation or panretinal photocoagulation (PRP). Panretinal photocoagulation is performed by placing multiple burns in the peripheral part of the retina. Usually, about 1,000 to 1,500 burns are placed in the periphery of the eye.

When will the treatment start?

In addition to monitoring the development of macular edema, your eye doctor checks for the development of neovascularization. You can wait a few days or weeks to have panretinal photocoagulation performed if the neovascularization is not severe. If there is extreme neovascularization and the eye has high-risk characteristics, scatter laser surgery probably should not be delayed.

In the majority of instances, PRP is performed in cases of moderate neovascularization. Sometimes, depending on the judgment of your ophthalmologist, PRP is also indicated when there is growth of new blood vessels in the front of the eyes (rubeosis). Often, rubeosis is also associated with glaucoma. In this situation, PRP should usually be performed without delay. Occasionally, the development of proliferative diabetic retinopathy can be quite rapid. Many studies have shown that scatter laser photocoagulation should be performed when there is significant retinopathy.

What is the procedure like?

First, pupils are dilated. Just as in focal laser treatment, scatter photocoagulation is performed with the slit lamp microscope, using a contact lens to stabilize the eye and to facilitate the surgery. After placement of the lens, between 1,000 and 2,000 burns are made. These laser burns are usually placed in the periphery of the retina. This operation is less delicate than focal laser photocoagulation. The procedure takes about thirty minutes to one hour.

The majority of patients do not feel pain, but many feel a mild discomfort akin to a sharp sensation. Usually, discomfort is felt when burns are placed close to a nerve. If you feel some discomfort, tell your ophthalmologist; he or she may then treat another area farther away from the nerves. Occasionally, patients feel more pain than they can tolerate. In these instances, a numbing injection can be given behind the eyes. This injection is called a retrobulbar block. This injection is very safe, but in rare instances, there are complications. These are listed in Table 5.1. In addition to the risks listed, there is a very small risk of retrobulbar hemorrhage, or bleeding into the eye socket. This is a very rare complication, but it may require emergency surgery to release the blood.

What are the benefits of PRP?

Untreated neovascularization and proliferative diabetic retinopathy often lead to such severe visual loss that you cannot see the big "E" on the Snellen chart at 10 feet. This is truly significant vision loss. Fortunately, panretinal laser photocoagulation is very effective for treatment of

ROBERT
"Anesthesia for laser surgery"

Robert is a fifty-two-year-old electrician who came to me after a vitreous hemorrhage in the left eye. He had had diabetes for about twelve years, but said that his blood sugar level has been under pretty good control. When I examined him, I found he had proliferative diabetic retinopathy in both eyes. It appeared that he needed scatter laser photocoagulation.

We discussed the risks and benefits of laser surgery and he agreed. When we first started treatment, Robert was feeling every burn the laser was making. I would reduce the power, but then I did not see the right reaction on the retina. In general, we put in between 1,200 and 1,400 burns per eye in two sessions. However, after only about 150 burns, we had to stop, because he was having too much discomfort.

Usually when a patient is having discomfort from the laser, I offer them an injection to numb the eye. This injection, called retrobulbar anesthesia, requires putting a needle behind the eyeball to place the anesthetic. Robert declined the injection; he was concerned about pain from the injection and also the risk of bleeding behind the eye. Robert considered his options and thought that his low pain tolerance was related to poor sleep from the previous night. He asked to have his laser surgery rescheduled.

When Robert returned, he was still feeling the same discomfort. I offered the injection again and he agreed. After the injection, Robert felt no pain or discomfort. He remarked to me that he will never have laser surgery again without the injection. He told me that the apprehension was much worse than the injection, while the pain from the laser was much worse than he could have guessed. If you feel more discomfort from the laser than you can tolerate, please be sure to ask your doctor for an injection.

proliferative diabetic retinopathy. The Diabetic Retinopathy Study (DRS) showed that treatment provided a 60 percent reduction in the risk of severe visual loss.

What are the risks and side effects of PRP?

Scatter laser surgery is very safe. The burns are made in the peripheral portion of the retina and not in the central fovea. The peripheral retina is important for peripheral and night vision. After panretinal photocoagulation, some individuals notice a constriction of the peripheral vision and some dimunition of night vision. Another side effect is worsening of macular edema and a subsequent decrease in vision. Similar to focal laser treatment, scatter laser surgery does not improve vision. Scatter laser surgery is done to prevent loss of vision. Some vision may have to be sacrificed in order to avoid greater losses of vision. Multiple studies have confirmed that even those patients who have some loss of vision from surgery would have lost much more vision if they had not had the procedure. Other side effects include worsening of scar tissue contraction

YURI
"Experimental treatment"

My wife's hairdresser told her in casual conversation that her husband Yuri had diabetes and decreased vision. My wife inquired about his medical care and found out that Yuri had seen several ophthalmologists but had refused treatment. Apparently, Yuri wanted to receive only experimental treatments. Because I was practicing in the Clinical Trials Branch of the National Eye Institute, National Institutes of Health (NIH) at that time, Yuri agreed to come see me.

Yuri was a fifty-year-old man who was diagnosed with diabetes fifteen years back when he was still living in the Soviet Union. He appeared slim and a little bit pale. I was concerned that he might also be anemic; many patients with diabetes also have anemia. He told me that he was seeing me to find out what experimental treatments were available for diabetic retinopathy. He emphasized that he did not want laser treatment and wanted only experimental treatments. I told him that we had a number of studies ongoing, but that I needed to examine him to determine for which studies he would qualify.

I proceeded to examine him and found that his vision was 20/200 on the right eye and 20/70 on the left. His pressures were normal. I dilated both of his pupils so that I could examine the inside of his eyes. He had severe macular edema in both eyes. I told him that laser treatment for macular edema is very effective. It can slow the loss of vision. He had lost a lot of vision in both eyes; the visual loss in the right was greater than in the left, but he still had a lot of vision left and therefore a lot of vision to lose. I told him that laser treatment had already been shown in clinical trials to be effective for macular edema, that the treatment was not uncomfortable, and that it could be done in the office. I went over the risks of laser surgery and also told him he had a 50 percent chance of losing an additional half of his vision if he chose not to have the laser surgery. I made drawings about the retina and spent a great deal of time with him.

After about fifteen minutes of explanation, he told me that he did not want to have the laser. He said that he did not believe in the principle of the laser, because it works by making tiny burns on the retina and he did not believe in destroying tissue. I told him that I, too, did not like damaging the retina. However, I told him that despite the seemingly destructive approach of the laser, it has been proven to be effective in slowing down visual loss. After another fifteen minutes, I still was not able to convince him to have the laser treatment. Yuri insisted on waiting until a therapy was available that was effective without making burns on the retina. I tried to convince him not to wait, because once vision is lost in diabetic retinopathy, it does not return. However, I was not successful. Yuri finally left and said that he would take his chances. He did promise to return in three months for a reevaluation, but he never came back.

I tried to convince Yuri not to worry about the actions of the laser. Although it is not a pill, and is considered surgery, laser treatment is very effective.

and temporary detachment of the retina by fluid (serous retinal detachment). Preventing a retinal detachment from scar tissue is another goal of scatter laser surgery. Serous retinal detachment is not desirable, of course, but fortunately, this kind of retinal detachment is temporary and has few long-term consequences.

One other consideration with laser surgery is that anxiety about the procedure or its discomfort may cause you to have low blood sugar. If you feel signs of low blood sugar, tell your ophthalmologist or nurse so that you can be treated appropriately.

Are there foods, drugs, or activities I should avoid after I receive this treatment?

There is no food or drug that you should avoid. There are also no activities that you should refrain from doing. However, you should continue your diabetic diet and your medications. You can continue to take all medications before and after laser surgery.

Are there other treatments besides PRP?

At present, there is no other procedure that has less risk than PRP for proliferative diabetic retinopathy. Vitrectomy surgery, which will be discussed later in this chapter, can be performed, but it has greater risks. There are no medications that are effective in treating neovascularization. As we discuss in Chapter 6, good control of your blood sugar will help prevent proliferative diabetic retinopathy in the first place. Once proliferative diabetic retinopathy develops, however, the only effective treatment is PRP.

Treatment of Vitreous Hemorrhage

One of the complications of neovascularization and proliferative diabetic retinopathy is bleeding from the new blood vessels. Normally, the hollow part of the eyeball is filled with a clear, transparent, jellylike substance called the vitreous. The vitreous is a structure that was necessary for early eye growth, but once the eye has reached maturity, the vitreous no longer is necessary. The problem with the vitreous is that it can contract with age and pull on the new blood vessels. This pulling can create a small hole in the new blood vessels, causing them to break. A break in the blood vessel will lead to bleeding into the vitreous. Blood in the eye is usually absorbed by the body. However, in the vitreous, the absorption can take a long time. Blood in the jellylike vitreous is not freely mobile; it is suspended and takes a long time to settle out. Trying to judge how long this will take is like asking how long it would take for the fruit in a bowl of Jell-O to settle to the bottom.

The treatment for vitreous hemorrhage is observation. Most hemorrhages eventually settle out. The settling process can take anywhere from one week to one year. However, in some situations, the treatment for the vitreous hemorrhage is surgical removal of the blood by vitrectomy surgery.

When is vitrectomy surgery necessary?

Vitrectomy surgery should be performed if your doctor feels that PRP needs to be performed, but she or he cannot see through the blood to perform the surgery. Vitrectomy surgery also should be performed if you have waited a while for the blood to clear and it has not done so on its own. Finally, if the retina is detached behind the blood, your doctor will likely recommend vitrectomy surgery to remove the blood and fix the detached retina.

What is vitrectomy surgery?

Vitrectomy surgery is performed in the operating room. A hospital stay is usually not required. Either local or general anesthesia is used. The goal of the procedure is to remove the blood along with any vitreous that is pulling on the new blood vessels. To accomplish this goal, three tiny openings are made into the eye (see Figure 5.4). A light source is placed in one so that the structures inside the eye are visible. A cutting suction needle is then placed into the

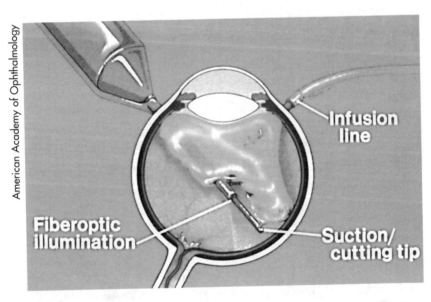

Figure 5.4 Schematic showing instruments in the eye demonstrating vitrectomy surgery

eye through the second opening to cut and remove the blood clots and vitreous. The third opening is for placement of a pipe that puts back clear fluid to replace the vitreous and the blood that is removed. After removing the blood, scar tissue is also removed. This reduces the likelihood of bleeding in the future and also reduces the chances of retinal detachment from contracture of the scar tissue. The operation takes from one to six hours, depending on how difficult it is to remove the scar tissue from the retina.

After the surgery, a patch is usually placed. The next morning, the patch is removed. It can take a bit of time for vision to return as the eye starts to heal. A few patients have rapid return of vision, but the majority have their best vision from three to six months after surgery. Three medications are usually used after the surgery (see Chapter 4).

What anesthesia is used?

Vitrectomy surgery can be done under local or general anesthesia. In local anesthesia the eye is numbed with an injection of anesthetic behind the eye (retrobulbar block). The anesthesiologist, a doctor who specializes in keeping surgery patients comfortable, will give you medication to help you forget the shot and make you sleepy during the surgery.

General anesthesia means you will be put to sleep during the procedure. What type of anesthesia to choose should be discussed with your doctor. Usually, if you can lie still for about one and a half hours and the surgery can be performed in that amount of time, local anesthesia can be used. If you do not think you can lay still for that long or your doctor feels that the surgery will take longer, general anesthesia would be preferable.

What are the benefits of vitrectomy surgery?

Benefits depend on the reason for the surgery. If vitrectomy surgery is performed to remove the blood to allow laser treatment, the operation is quite effective—the success rate is over 90 percent.

However, outcomes are a bit poorer when one looks at visual improvement after surgery. In general, the blood can be removed without difficulty. However, there is a significant chance that rebleeding will occur. In addition, the benefit of vitrectomy surgery appears to be greater for younger individuals than for older ones. There are several explanations for this. One is that in older patients, the macula, the very center of the retina, may have undergone some age-related changes that limit its visual potential. Cataracts also tend to develop following vitrectomy surgery. It may be that in older persons, the formation of cataracts occurs sooner, thus reducing the chance of better vision. Whatever the reason, your doctor is less likely to recommend vitrectomy surgery if you are older.

The success of vitrectomy surgery for vitreous hemorrhage and retinal detachment varies depending on the duration and extent of the detachment, the underlying health of the retina itself, and the extent of any cataract.

What are the risks of vitrectomy surgery?

Operations that involve putting instruments inside the eye are fundamentally different from those involving the laser that are done in the office. Vitrectomy operations have a higher risk of serious complications.

Table 5.1 lists the risks of vitrectomy surgery. However, considering these risks requires some perspective. In general, nothing is risk free in life, even simple things that we take for granted. For example, when you cross the street, there are lots of risks. You could trip and sprain your ankle when you step off the sidewalk. A car or a truck could come careening around the corner and strike you. Even if the car does not strike you and only comes close, the emotional stress could give you a heart attack. Given all these risks, most of us still cross the street. We do it because the risk of these events is quite small and the benefit of getting where we want to go is much greater. Similarly, surgery is not without risks, but when it is recommended, the benefit usually outweighs the risks. Table 5.1 should be viewed with this in mind.

With any surgery, there is always the chance that the problem cannot be fixed. This risk is what we call failure to accomplish intent of surgery. Sometimes when this happens, additional surgery might be indicated. At other times, the surgeon may tell you that more surgery would not be helpful.

Because instruments are put inside the eye for this operation, there is a risk that they can damage the retina. The instruments can also pull on the vitreous, which is attached to the retina. This pulling can lead to retinal detachment, a serious complication. More surgery might need to be performed, but additional surgery may not fix the problem. Retinal detachment in a patient with diabetes is a serious situation.

One common side effect of vitrectomy surgery is the development of a cataract. As we discussed in Chapter 2, a cataract is a cloudy lens. Vitrectomy surgery tends to speed up the formation of cataract. If a cataract develops, another operation might need to be done to remove the cataract and put in an implant.

Serious infection that develops inside the eye following surgery is not common. It occurs in less than 1 in 1,000 cases. However, eyes that develop this infection (endophthalmitis) are seriously injured. This kind of infection, inside the eye, is different from infection that occurs on the outside of the eye, such as pinkeye, or conjunctivitis. Once infection develops inside the eye, very little vision is recovered even if the infection is controlled. Pinkeye, or infection outside the eye, rarely causes vision loss.

There is also a risk of serious bleeding at the time of surgery. The risk is not high, but the consequences from this complication are quite severe. The risk of serious bleeding, however, is less than 1 in 1,000.

Are there foods, drugs, or activities I should avoid before or after the surgery?

Your doctor may want you to avoid eating or drinking anything for twelve hours before the operation. This will ensure that you have an empty stomach, so that your stomach contents do not accidentally spill into your lungs during the surgery. If your doctor asks you not to eat or drink, you may want to ask whether you should take your medications. In general, important medications probably should be taken with a small sip of water. Usually, the anesthesiologist or your diabetes doctor will let you know which medications you should take before surgery. Your insulin dose will probably be reduced by half.

There are no food or drug restrictions after the surgery.

There are no absolute restrictions on activities. Your doctor may ask you to avoid contact sports, heavy lifting, stooping, or bending. He may ask you to sleep on several pillows. Wearing glasses to protect your repaired eye or a shield at bedtime may be encouraged. However, many patients who have had major surgery take off several days or weeks to recover. The exact recovery period depends on you and your doctor. Some people go back to work the very next day. Those who undergo a long operation under general anesthesia may want to take longer.

Are there other treatments available?

Blood in the vitreous can be absorbed by the body. Oftentimes, the blood takes six months to a year before it goes away. However, if fresh bleeding occurs while you are waiting for the first hemorrhage to clear, you would have to wait an additional six months from the last bleeding episode. A decision to have vitrectomy surgery depends on how long one can or wants to wait. If there is not an urgent need to perform laser surgery on the retina, and if the patient can see well out of the other eye, observation is a real alternative. However, if panretinal photocoagulation is necessary, there is no other choice but to remove the blood and perform laser treatment.

Treatment of Retinal Detachment

The retina is the portion of the eye that is sensitive to light. If the eye is a camera, think of it as the "film." Normally, the retina lines the inside of the eyeball. Under certain circumstances, the retina separates from the inside of the eyeball (see Figure 5.5). When this happens, it is called a retinal detachment. Retinal detachment can occur for a variety of reasons. In diabetes, retinal detachment usually occurs because of scar tissue that develops from neovascularization and contracts.

Retinal detachment is not good for the functioning of the eye. When the retina is separated from the eye wall, the rod and cone layer of the retina loses its supply of nutrients. Starved, the photoreceptors die and the retina functions poorly. People with this condition often notice that they have a nonseeing area in the portion of their vision occupied by the retinal detachment. Most retinal detachments do not improve by themselves. The only way to restore function is to repair the retinal detachment.

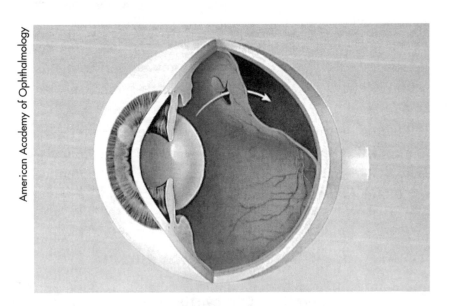

American Academy of Ophthalmology

Figure 5.5 Schematic of the eye showing retinal detachment. The arrow shows fluid entering a retinal tear causing retinal detachment.

When should retinal detachment surgery be performed?

If the retinal detachment has caused loss of vision or is threatening vision, almost all eye doctors recommend surgery to repair it. As discussed, a detached retina does not function properly, and there is very little chance that the retina will fix itself.

If vision is lost due to a retinal detachment, fixing the detachment does not guarantee that the vision will return. Some vision will come back, but not all of it. How much vision will come back depends on how long the retina is detached and what portion of it is detached. If the center of the retina, the macula, is detached, the chance of restoring good vision is less. The macula is the most sensitive portion of the retina. Any separation of the macula from the eye wall will lead to some irreversible vision loss. It is much better to fix a retinal detachment before the central macula detaches. If the macula remains attached, the prognosis for vision loss is significantly diminished.

Retinal detachments of long standing can also be more difficult to fix. Once the retina loses its blood supply, it often begins to lose substance (atrophy). When the retina thins out, the surgery becomes more difficult. Fixing a detachment that has just happened is easier than fixing one that has developed scar tissue over many months or years. Removing scar tissue from thin retina is like removing bubblegum from tissue paper.

If your doctor recommends surgery, ask how long you can safely wait before further vision loss ensues. In certain situations, your eye doctor may want to operate immediately, that very day. The reason for this urgency is to prevent the macula from detaching.

How is a retinal detachment repaired?

There are several ways to fix a retinal detachment. Because it results from scar tissue pulling on the retina, surgery involves either removing the scar tissue or minimizing the amount of pulling on the retina with a scleral buckle. A scleral buckle supports the eye; it is a belt around the outside of the eye so that the separated retina is pushed back against the eye wall.

The operation to remove the scar tissue from the inside of the eye involves first removing the vitreous and then removing the scar. Like surgery for a vitreous hemorrhage, the first part of the operation is removal of the vitreous with a vitrectomy. After the vitreous is removed, the scar tissue is then peeled from the retina. This portion of the surgery is quite difficult. The retina is a very delicate part of the eye and removing scar tissue from its surface often can lead to rips in the retina. If and when this occurs, these tears will need to be repaired. Laser burns are placed to seal the holes and gas is injected inside the eye to "reinflate" the retina.

With certain detachments, gas is injected into the eye at the end of the vitrectomy operation. Gas is placed into the eye to cover any holes in the retina. Without gas injection, fluid that is normally present in the eye would pass freely through the holes and cause a redetachment of the retina. When gas is present, fluid is displaced from the area of the holes, preventing it from entering. Depending on how long your doctor feels that the gas is needed, he may inject gas that lasts twenty-four hours (air), two weeks (sulfur hexafluoride gas), and six weeks (C_3F_8 gas). Rarely, a gas or substance is needed to displace fluid indefinitely from a part of the retina. In such circumstances, the doctor will inject silicone oil instead. It acts exactly the same way, except that the eye cannot resorb it like gas. When the silicone oil has done its job, it requires removal with another operation.

The alternate procedure to repair retinal detachment is to suture a piece of silicone rubber to the outside of the eye to push the eye wall against the lifted-off retina. The eye is indented in the middle like an hourglass. This operation is called a scleral buckle. The silicone that is placed around the eye is inert and can stay around the eye for the rest of your life. No one who meets you will ever know that you had a scleral buckle placed around your eye. It is not visible.

What anesthesia is used?

Retinal detachment surgery can be done under local or general anesthesia. Again, this choice should be discussed with your doctor. If you can lie still for about one and a half hours and the surgery can be performed in that amount of time, local anesthesia can be used. However, if you have claustrophobia, cannot lay still for long, or your doctor feels that the surgery will take longer than that, general anesthesia would be preferable.

What are the benefits of retinal detachment surgery?

A detached retina will not function. Reattaching the retina will lead to the resumption of function. If the detachment is recent and the macula was not detached before surgery, then reattaching the retina can lead to the return of useful vision. However, if the detachment is long standing, the chance of being able to fix the retina is reduced. If the macula was detached, returning the detached macula to its original position will not restore all vision.

What are the risks and side effects associated with this procedure?

The risks of retinal detachment surgery are listed in Table 5.1. Unlike laser surgery or cataract surgery, vitrectomy and retina surgery have the highest chance of failure with the first operation. With retinal detachment, there is more chance that additional surgery will be needed to repair it.

There is also a risk that the initial surgery may cause retinal tears that can lead to bigger retinal detachments. Sometimes, the surgery can cause a detachment that is not fixable. This is an unfortunate complication, but it is a risk of the surgery.

During the retinal detachment operation, the "skin" on the cornea (corneal epithelium) may need to be removed to permit better visualization. If this occurs, there will be a gritty sensation in the eye after the surgery until the "skin" heals. The healing process can take days and, for diabetics, weeks. Another side effect of this missing epithelium is that vision will be decreased until it heals.

Are there foods, drugs, or activities I should avoid after vitrectomy or retinal surgery?

Your doctor may want you to avoid eating or drinking anything for twelve hours before the operation, so that your stomach contents do not accidentally spill into your lungs during the surgery. If your doctor asks you not to eat or drink, ask whether you should take your medications. In general, important medications probably should be taken with a small sip of water. Your insulin dose will probably be reduced by half.

There are no restrictions following most retinal detachment repair operations. In general, you should try to rest after retinal surgery. There is no set time that everyone should rest. You should use good judgment. If after a few minutes of activity, your treated eye tends to ache, you may want to rest more. Many patients rest four to six weeks before returning to work, while other patients wait only several days after surgery.

The patch placed after surgery should be kept dry for at least twenty-four hours. Your doctor may instruct you to remove the patch and start putting some drops in your eyes the morning following surgery, or she or he may ask you to leave the patch in place until your first visit. During the first week after surgery, be extra careful and try to avoid splashing water or other substances into the eye.

Sometimes during this surgery, a gas bubble or air is injected into the eye to ensure that the retina has the highest likelihood of being repaired. If a gas bubble is in the eye, you should avoid air travel or traveling to high altitudes. High altitudes may cause the gas bubble to increase in size. This causes high pressure in the eye, which can then cause glaucoma and may lead to pain and vision loss. Your doctor may also instruct you to lie in a position that will improve the effectiveness of the bubble. If gas is injected, you will probably be asked to remain face-down for the duration of the gas bubble. This position is used because gas bubbles behave in only one way—they rise up. Most of the time, gas is injected for holes in the middle of the eye. To get the gas there, you have to rotate your head toward the ground. When you stand or sit up, the gas bubble stays in the same place, but you would have moved the eye away from the gas bubble. Remaining face-down means that you sleep face-down, eat face-down, go to the bathroom face-down, and walk around face-down; you have to be in this position all the time. The success of operations that use gas often depends on the patient's ability to comply with this twenty-four-hour positioning for weeks on end.

What is the healing time?

Healing time varies from patient to patient. It may be very difficult for the patient to tell how the retina is healing. The best way to gauge this is to attend regular follow-up appointments with your doctor and ask how the healing is progressing. The main worry with retinal detachment surgery is that the retina will redetach despite a previously successful operation. The longer the retina stays attached after surgery, the more likely that it will stay attached permanently. In general, retina specialists tend to wait about three months before the surgery is considered successful. If you have had your retina detachment repaired, your doctor will follow you closely for three months, and possibly take you back to surgery again during that time if your retina has redetached. Your doctor may encourage you to change your glasses prescription, but he or she will likely wait a full three months after surgery to ensure that your retina is stable.

Are other treatments available?

We have discussed the two basic options for managing detached retinas. Under certain circumstances, a gas bubble may be injected to repair certain kinds of retinal detachments. This kind of treatment (pneumatic retinopexy) is not usually effective for treating retinal detachments from diabetic retinopathy. However, persons with diabetes may develop this special kind of retinal detachment, distinct from diabetes, that can be fixed with the injection of a gas bubble.

Before, During, and After Surgery

1. Make sure you understand the risks and benefits of the surgery. Here are some questions you may want to ask your ophthalmologist:

- ❖ Why do you think surgery is the best treatment for my condition?
- ❖ What kind of surgery do you recommend for my condition, and why?
- ❖ Are there other treatment options I should consider?
- ❖ What do you think might happen if I don't have the surgery?
- ❖ Do you think I am likely to need further treatment after the surgery (for example, further surgery)?
- ❖ What change should I expect in my condition after surgery?
- ❖ What kind of anesthesia will you use for my surgery?
- ❖ Where will my surgery take place?
- ❖ When will my surgery take place?
- ❖ Approximately how long will my surgery take?
- ❖ Should I discontinue any of my medications prior to surgery? If so, how long before my surgery should I stop taking them?
- ❖ Can I eat prior to my surgery?

You might find it helpful to write down your questions prior to your office visit, or to take notes during your appointment. This can help ensure that you understand everything your ophthalmologist discusses with you.

2. If you have medical insurance, you should find out if your policy will cover your surgery, and how much, if anything, you should expect to pay out of pocket.

3. Most importantly, don't be afraid to ask your ophthalmologist questions. If you have any concerns, now is the time to discuss them with your doctor.

The day of your surgery

1. If you've been told not to eat before surgery, it is very important to follow that instruction. It can be dangerous to eat prior to undergoing some kinds of anesthesia.

2. Most hospitals and outpatient facilities recommend you leave valuables, such as money or jewelry, at home. You may not be allowed to take those items into the procedure room.

3. If you are having your procedure in a hospital or outpatient surgery facility, make sure you get there in time to fill out any registration forms that may be required.

What will happen the day of surgery?

❖ After you have registered or checked in, you may go to a waiting room or area prior to your surgery. You may be asked to change into a patient gown for your surgery. Depending on the kind of anesthesia you and your doctor selected for your procedure, an anesthesiologist may spend a few minutes talking with you to make sure it is the safest kind for you, and to answer any additional questions.

❖ In the procedure room, you may be asked to sit in a special chair or lie on a table, depending on what kind of surgery you are having.

❖ Your ophthalmologist or an assistant will probably put drops in your eyes to numb them. This is the only anesthesia necessary for some patients having laser surgery. He or she may also give you an injection to help numb the whole area around your eye. This usually involves a minimum of discomfort.

❖ If you and your ophthalmologist decide you need seda-
tion—medication to make you less anxious—you may be
given an injection or have an intravenous line (i.v.) placed in
your arm. (This means a small needle will be placed in your
arm and connected to some tubing and a bag of sterile solution and medication.) This usually doesn't hurt any more than
getting a shot or giving blood.

❖ If your surgery is a laser procedure, you will be seated in
a special chair in front of the laser instruments while the surgeon uses a beam of laser light to perform the procedure.

❖ If you are having a vitrectomy, the ophthalmologist or the
assistant will place sterile drapes around your eye. You won't be
able to feel the surgery, or see it with the eye being repaired.

❖ The time your surgery takes depends on many factors, such
as your eye structure and the kind of surgery being performed.

After your surgery
After your surgery, the ophthalmologist or assistant may
put more drops in your eyes. You may be given medication for discomfort. You might need to wear an eye
patch to protect the eye. You will probably have to wait
for a period after your surgery to make sure it's safe for
you to return home. You may have to stay a little longer
if you've been sedated.

1. Prior to leaving, you should be given instructions about:
❖ medications—when you should start taking them,
and how often
❖ what to expect in the next few hours or days—for
example, how much discomfort or swelling you
may have

- ❖ what signs to look for that might indicate infection or other problems
- ❖ what activities you must refrain from, and for how long
- ❖ when you should return to the ophthalmologist for follow-up
- ❖ how to contact your ophthalmologist if you have later questions or concerns

2. If you have any other questions or concerns at this time, ask your ophthalmologist or the assistant or nurse before you leave.

3. Make sure you have a friend or family member to drive you home after your procedure. You may have an eye patch, or feel slightly groggy after your surgery.

4. Make sure you understand your ophthalmologist's instructions and follow them carefully. This will help ensure a speedy recovery and good outcome.

5. Keep your follow-up appointment(s), even if you have no sutures (stitches) to remove and are experiencing no complications.

6. Above all, take care of yourself and your eyes. Maintain a healthy diet and get regular exercise. Keep your blood sugar under good control. Wear sunglasses with adequate UV protection when you're in the sun, and make sure your eyes are protected when you play sports or use heavy machinery.

6

Self-Monitoring, Glucose Control, and Prevention

Glucose control is the basis of diabetes management, and sometimes it can be very frustrating. For diabetics, maintaining close-to-normal sugar means a constant balancing act between diet, exercise, and insulin use. For many, it means frequent glucose monitoring and insulin adjustments. Sometimes you can do all the right things and your sugar still acts "crazy." Even with a well-regulated routine, stress, illness, or alcohol consumption can throw the balance into the danger zone.

Since the discovery of insulin in 1921, advances in diabetes care continue to occur; however, we have not yet discovered a way to duplicate the actions of the pancreas with perfection. We must rely on checking sugars with commercial monitors and injecting insulin in response. These portable systems, called glucometers, enable diabetics to measure their blood glucose with great accuracy and adjust their insulin appropriately. More recently, insulin pumps allow diabetics even more control of their glucose levels by administering a continuous amount of a small dose of basal insulin and supplementing this with occasional boluses (larger doses) depending on food intake.

For years, medical researchers speculated that strict glucose control might reduce the risk of complications from diabetes. Diabetics developed vision loss, kidney disease, neuropathy (numbness in their hands and feet), and seemed to have heart attacks at an earlier age. Today, thanks to a major national study, we know that tight glucose control does reduce the risk of complications. This study, involving twenty-seven centers across the country, was called the Diabetes Control and Complications Trial (DCCT) and helped us understand the importance of glucose control. It is the basis on which we recommend to our patients the importance of glucose control to prevent blindness from diabetic retinopathy.

Will controlling my sugars prevent me from going blind?

Our patients worry about going blind from their diabetes. Most of our patients are referred to us from general ophthalmologists and optometrists who see some form of diabetic retinopathy in their eyes. One of the most common questions we are asked is, "Am I going to go blind from my diabetes?" Diabetics and family members want to know what can be done for the diabetic retinopathy and how they can slow or prevent diabetes from affecting the eyesight.

In general, controlling your diabetes with the help of your internist and careful ophthalmology screening and follow-up will prevent blindness.

Not every patient has the same severity of diabetes.

Some diabetics are what we call "brittle." This means that it is very difficult for them to control their diabetes. Their blood sugar fluctuates more easily. Other people are told that they just have a "touch of sugar" and have been asked to watch their diets. It is important to be aware that diabetes can affect individual people differently. The program recommended for you to manage your diabetes may be different than the one implemented for your next-door neighbor.

What is self-monitoring?

Self-monitoring means that you use a glucose meter (one of many name brands) to check your blood sugar by yourself. Glucose meters can be obtained through your local hospital's diabetic coordinator or diabetic educator. They can also be purchased at your local pharmacy without a prescription.

To check your own blood sugar with a glucose meter, first wash your hands. A sterile lancet enclosed in the monitoring kit is used to prick a finger. A drop of blood is squeezed onto a test strip. The test strip is inserted into the glucose meter and a number will appear, indicating your blood sugar level. A normal blood sugar is less than 110 milligrams.

Some patients with vision loss from diabetes confide that they can't read the monitor. They are unable to test their sugars unless a family member is around to read it for them. Now, I ask all my patients about self-monitoring and our office helps teach our diabetics how to use a monitor if they wish to learn. There are talking glucose monitors, like talking blood pressure monitors, and there are magnifiers that will make the display easier to see. If you are having trouble reading the monitor, make sure you tell your doctor so that he or she can help you.

Is there a way to check your blood sugar that doesn't involve a finger prick?

No reliable "non-stick" method yet exists. There has been a lot of hype about noninvasive blood glucose meters which use infrared spectroscopy to produce a signature of glucose or detect the glucose level through a skin sensor; however, they need further development.

Which diabetics should check their own blood sugars?

Your doctor will tell you whether to self-monitor. In general, anyone taking insulin should know how to check glucose and adjust the insulin dose based on a low or high sugar.

How was the national study done which advocated glucose control?

The DCCT was a large study, involving twenty-seven centers throughout the country, which tested the theory that the complications of diabetes mellitus are related to high glucose concentration in the blood. Both types of diabetes can result in complications which involve tissue damage, but only Type I diabetics were included in this study. The tissues most commonly damaged are the eyes, kidneys, and nerves. The study compared two groups of Type I diabetics who monitored their glucose differently in order to answer the question, "Can diabetic complications be prevented or their development slowed if better control of glucose levels could be achieved?"

The study lasted seven years and compared two groups of patients with Type I diabetics. The first group received conventional, or standard treatment and the second group received intensive treatment. The goal of the standard treatment group was clinical well-being; the goal of the intensive treatment group was normalization of blood glucose.

Standard therapy: "Clinical well-being" means avoiding the symptoms that poorly controlled diabetics get. Poorly controlled diabetics have frequent urination, increased thirst, and frequent or severe low blood sugar. Children (older than thirteen) were also included in this group and were weighed and measured to avoid growth failure. Insulin was administered one or two times daily. Nutritional counseling was provided to achieve the above goals.

With a special test, hemoglobin A_{1c} (HbA_{1c}) levels were measured every three months. This test is a doctor's way of knowing how well controlled sugars have been in the previous three months without actually seeing a record of every high and low sugar. If this test was higher than 13 percent (normal is less than 6 percent in nondiabetics), then the insulin dose was changed.

Intensive therapy: The goal of this group was to obtain normal blood glucose levels. This approach involved multiple doses of regular insulin. Also, all patients received a baseline dose of either intermediate or long-acting insulin or a continuous insulin infusion pump, which constantly delivers insulin in tiny doses.

The specific glucose goals were as follows: before meals 70–120 mg/dl, two hours after a meal <180 mg/dl, and a 3:00 A.M. glucose of >65 mg/dl. The diabetes team taught patients to monitor their blood glucose at appropriate times and to administer their insulin in the right amount at the right times. The hemoglobin A_{1c} was measured monthly in this group to provide frequent feedback; the goal was less than 6 percent (upper limit of normal in nondiabetics).

The intensive treatment group received monthly encouragement from members of the diabetes team (diabetes nurse educators, dietitians, behavioral scientists, and physicians). The team members were available twenty-four hours a day and consultation could take place at any time.

What did this study conclude?

In the intensively treated group, a 60 percent reduction in the risk of developing microvascular (tiny blood vessel) complications—diabetic retinopathy (the eyes), nephropathy (the kidneys), and neuropathy (the nerves)— occurred. Intensive treatment slowed both the onset of these complications and the rate of progression. The benefit of treatment was seen among all ages in the study regardless of gender or duration of diabetes.

What is glucose control?

"Control" means keeping the level of your sugar close to normal. It requires the right balance between the food you eat (increases blood sugar), the amount of exercise you do (lowers blood sugar), and the amount of insulin you take (lowers blood sugar). Control also means that you avoid episodes of low sugar and high sugar. For children, it also means normal growth and development.

What is tight control, and how was this measured in the DCCT?

The term *tight control* is used to indicate blood glucose levels equal to or better than those achieved by the intensively treated group. A measure of the success of glucose control is the hemoglobin A_{1c} level, or glycated hemoglobin level. As discussed, this is a test of blood glucose concentration over a three-month period. A high percentage of HbA_{1c} indicates poor control whereas a low percentage indicates good control.

The goal of intensive therapy is to achieve as close to normal blood glucose as possible. This is accomplished either with insulin pumps or with four or more injections of insulin daily, adjusting the insulin dose based on frequent (up to seven times daily) home blood glucose monitoring. Patients who entered the study had, on average, a glycosolated hemoglobin (HgA_{1c}) at about 9.0 and stayed the same when randomized to standard therapy, while patients receiving intensive therapy reduced their HgA_{1c} about 20 percent to 7.2 percent and maintained this level throughout the study.

What target level of glucose control should I aim for?

Other factors than glucose control, such as genetics, influence the risk of complications. Nevertheless, patients should aim for the best level of glucose control they can achieve without placing themselves at undue risk of hypo-glycemia or other hazards associated with tight control.

Treatment of your diabetes needs to be individualized after consulting with your doctor. If the Type I patient is intellectually, emotionally, physically, and financially able to attempt tight control, and if a health care team is available to provide resources, guidance, and support, a reasonable goal is the average glucose level and HbA_{1c} levels obtained in the trial. The average glucose level was 155 mg/dl and the average HbA_{1c} level was 7.2 percent. In a nondiabetic, the average glucose is 110 mg/dl and the average HbA_{1c} level is ≤6 percent.

For those choosing tight control, is lifelong intensive treatment necessary?

In general, tight control for diabetics past puberty should be maintained for life. Increasing age or other illness (stroke, heart attack, or frequent low sugar which places the patient or others at severe risk) may require a change in diabetes management.

What complications of diabetes are prevented by tightly controlling sugars?

In the body, there are large and small blood vessels. Blood vessels carry blood from one place to another just like a garden hose carries water from the faucet to the yard. When blood flow is compromised, the tissues get sick. If someone steps on the garden hose, the plants get less water and might shrivel up.

One set of complications from poorly controlled

diabetes is designated microvascular or small blood vessel disease. Microvascular complications affect three tissues in the body: the eyes (retinopathy), the kidneys (nephropathy), and the nerves (neuropathy). These complications lead to visual loss, kidney failure, and multiple neurological symptoms including pain, burning sensation, impotence, and foot ulcers from loss of pain sensation in the feet.

A second set of complications is termed macrovascular or large blood vessel disease. Macrovascular disease is due to atherosclerotic complications or "hardening of the arteries," which results in less blood flow to the tissues. Complications from large blood vessel disease include angina or chest pain, heart attacks, strokes, and amputations. Diabetes is not the only process which contributes to large vessel disease; smoking, high blood pressure, and abnormal blood cholesterol levels are also risk factors.

Can tight control be dangerous? What are the symptoms of low blood sugar?

Yes, it can be. Low blood sugar and weight gain are the two risks present with tight control. In the DCCT, the intensive treatment group had a threefold risk of severe hypoglycemia than did the standard treatment group. Hypoglycemia is low blood sugar. Early symptoms of low blood sugar are nervousness, jitters or the shakes, confusion, dizziness, irritable mood, hunger, and sweatiness. If it isn't treated in time by eating or drinking sugar, serious hypoglycemia can cause one to pass out, or to develop coma and seizures, resulting in injury to the patient or to others.

The danger of hypoglycemia can be reduced by frequent monitoring and insulin adjustment, as well as changing the content and frequency of meals and snacks, and changing exercise patterns. Self-education and management training are very important if tight control is attempted. Hypoglycemia may have harmful effects on intellectual and psychological function in children, although these side effects were not seen in the DCCT. This study was limited to children older than age thirteen.

Weight gain also occurred in the intensively treated

ANNE
"Tight control with the pump"

Anne is a forty-two-year-old working mother of two children who developed gestational diabetes during her second pregnancy. She subsequently developed diabetes treated first with oral medications and, finally, insulin. Her insulin requirement was increasing and she had difficulty controlling her sugars despite frequent monitoring and insulin use. She had gained over 20 pounds since her last pregnancy and had mild nonproliferative diabetic retinopathy. She had frequent episodes of hypoglycemia and was terrified of another incident requiring someone's assistance. She wanted to be placed on the insulin pump; however, her doctor tried to dissuade her from using it. She sought out another physician, and she began to use an insulin pump. She was thrilled with the improved glucose control, the flexibility to eat when she wanted, and the fact that she had less hypoglycemic episodes. The insulin pump required that she use less insulin, so she gained less weight.

group. Insulin increases glucose uptake into the body's tissues. Weight gain can have emotional and medical consequences. The health care team can help monitor weight, adjust diet, and develop individual exercise programs to combat this side effect.

Use of the insulin pump (CSII, continuous simultaneous insulin infusion) reduces the total daily dose of insulin by 25 percent. Because this total dose is less, people attempting tight control tend to gain less weight than people using multiple daily injections. Also, hypoglycemic episodes occur less frequently with the insulin pump. Patients using the pump learn to count carbohydrates.

Can complications be avoided in Type II diabetics?

Because the same complications occur in Type II and Type I diabetics, there is no reason to think that the results of this study would not apply to both groups; the same or similar underlying disease mechanisms apply.

However, tight control may not be advisable in obese persons. Many Type II patients are also obese. Obesity is associated with insulin resistance; the body doesn't respond to the normal levels of insulin it has. The weight gain characteristic of intensive therapy could create a vicious cycle in Type II diabetics.

Weight Gain

Because of an increased occurrence of macrovascular disease in Type II diabetics, older patients may be more susceptible to serious consequences of hypoglycemia, including fainting, seizures, heart attack, stroke, and even death. Some doctors believe that the higher insulin doses required to overcome insulin resistance may be a factor in the development of high blood pressure, abnormal cholesterol levels, and atherosclerosis in Type II patients.

Treatment should be individualized. A new drug, Rezulin, or troglitazone, is being prescribed for people with insulin resistance with good success. Troglitazone increases insulin sensitivity. Rarely, this medication can cause liver damage. Your doctor will check your liver enzymes before you start the medication as well as periodically while you take the medication.

The results of the DCCT suggest that many otherwise healthy persons with Type II diabetes should strive to achieve tight control. Older age, significant heart disease, or history of stroke are reasons not to pursue tight control.

An eighty-eight-year-old woman was recently admitted to the hospital for a mild stroke. We were asked to examine her eyes because she had had diabetes for fourteen years. She told us she could see her bingo card without glasses and her lucky number was B13. She'd never had an eye problem in her life. Her vision was indeed excellent, and we noted only mild diabetic eye changes. Her only medication was Glucotrol, and she had never monitored her sugars on her own. Her daughter was fifty-two years old and also had diabetes. Her daughter took insulin and checked her sugars four times daily. The daughter wanted to know whether her mother might need to be on insulin to prevent another stroke and to prevent the diabetic eye disease from getting worse. Her elderly age, her history of stroke, the mild stage of her eye disease, and the fact that her sugars during her hospital stay ran between 120–140 mg/dl prompted her physician to not recommend tight control.

Whether or not tight control is pursued, risk factors for atherosclerosis should be minimized. Stopping smoking, lowering cholesterol and blood pressure, and losing weight can reduce the risk of macrovascular complications.

Does tight control reduce macrovascular complications?

Atherosclerosis occurs earlier in people with diabetes than it does in those without elevated blood glucose levels. It is reasonable to assume that tight control would reduce the risk of macrovascular complications.

Did the DCCT show that intensive treatment reduced the risk of retinopathy, vision loss, and ultimately blindness?

The study graded the spectrum of retinopathy in twenty-five steps from no retinopathy to severe proliferative retinopathy. A three-step change on the scale was considered a significant finding. In the intensively treated group, patients with no retinopathy at baseline showed a 76 percent reduction in risk of developing a significant change over a six-month time frame. In patients with mild to moderate retinopathy at baseline, there was a 54 percent reduction in the same endpoint. There was a 46 percent reduction in the development of severe nonproliferative or proliferative retinopathy. A 56 percent reduction in the need for laser surgery was also found in the group with mild to moderate retinopathy at baseline.

If blindness has already occurred, should tight control be pursued?

Tight control may not be recommended for patients who already have marked visual loss or end-stage renal disease. Patients with advanced complications were not entered into the trial, so no direct evidence is available to indicate that tight control in such patients is beneficial. Again, discussion with your diabetes doctor is very important.

One of my patients is legally blind from diabetic retinopathy and is on dialysis three times a week. He also has hypertension which is difficult to control and wears a cast over his left foot because of diabetic neuropathy and a foot ulcer. Tight control would not be especially beneficial for him, although he takes insulin and checks his sugar twice daily. He has difficulty maintaining his balance because of his vision and foot cast, and he is very nervous about having a low sugar reaction and falling. After careful discussion with his doctors, tight control was not recommended. Despite being legally blind, we still must examine his eyes frequently to prevent the development of glaucoma and to monitor for bleeding inside the eye.

If intensive treatment is not a realistic goal for me, should I still have an eye examination?

Absolutely. Having an eye examination by a trained ophthalmologist who can recognize early signs of diabetic retinopathy as well as potential serious problems is important to maintaining good vision. Timely diagnosis and treatment of retinopathy can reduce your risk of severe vision loss by more than 50 percent (see Chapter 3 on eye examinations and diabetes).

Are the results of the DCCT achievable for most people with diabetes?

In theory, the answer is yes. In reality, a great effort will be required to reproduce the results of the DCCT. The study group was young, generally healthy, and highly motivated. The professional personnel conducting the study were trained endocrinologists and diabetes educators in academic centers who were enthusiastic and meticulous in their management of the study patients. The intensively treated group received far more attention and services than are routinely available.

Broad implementation of intensive therapy will require expanded health care teams—diabetologists, diabetes educators, nutritionists, social workers—patient educational efforts, and an enhanced partnership between specialists such as ophthalmologists and primary care providers. The costs of implementing such a program will be substantial; however, cost-benefit studies have shown that reducing long-term complications will save on future medical costs, as well as improve the quality of life for diabetic patients.

Diabetes is a manageable disease if you accept that it is with you for the long haul. Learn to incorporate self-monitoring into your daily routine. Take the time to learn all you can about the disease, your treatment plan, and how to adjust your medications based upon illness, change in diet, and change in exercise.

What else can I do besides monitoring and tight control of blood sugar to prevent blindness?

Control your blood pressure and make sure your cholesterol is normal by seeing your doctor regularly. Most important to your eyes is to have them examined routinely even if your vision seems perfect.

7

Vision Loss

Diabetes mellitus is the leading cause of blindness among working-age Americans. The Early Treatment Diabetic Retinopathy Study (ETDRS) was the most recent National Institutes of Health study on diabetic retinopathy. The ETDRS studied 3,711 patients and followed them for an average of over five years. This study showed that the risk of severe visual loss is quite low with today's modern management of diabetic retinopathy. In this study, Dr. Fong and collaborators found that the most common causes of vision loss were vitreous hemorrhage, macular edema, macular/retinal detachment, and neovascular glaucoma.

Causes of Vision Loss

Vitreous Hemorrhage
Vitreous hemorrhage is bleeding into the normally clear interior of the eye. The area behind the lens and in front of the retina is called the vitreous cavity. Normally, this cavity

is filled with a jellylike substance called the vitreous. The vitreous does not fulfill any function in the adult eye. In the fetal eye, the vitreous is thought to provide pressure for normal eye growth and to act like a cushion to injury from the outside of the eye.

As we discussed in Chapter 2, diabetes leads to growth of new blood vessels, called neovascularization. The new blood vessels, once formed, are very susceptible to bleeding. Blood from these neovascular blood vessels collects in the vitreous cavity.

Blood in the vitreous cavity can go away by itself. If there is a lot of blood in the eye or if the blood obscures your doctor's view inside your eye, then surgery may be recommended. The operation is called a vitrectomy operation. In this operation, the blood and vitreous substance is removed and the eye is filled back with a balanced saline solution.

Macular Edema

The retina is the part of the eye that is sensitive to light; it can be thought of as the film of the eye. The very center of the retina is the macula. The macula is the part of the eye that gives you the sharpest vision. Without the macula, you would be legally blind, even if the rest of the eye was working properly. The macula is probably the most delicate part of the retina and the eye.

In diabetes, the blood vessels in the macula often become damaged and leak. Leakage leads to accumulation of fluid and material and is called edema. In other parts of the eye, leakage may be present, but not noticed. However, because the macula is so delicate, any disturbance of the structure in this area leads to changes in vision. Early on, patients with macular edema may only notice some distortion. However, over time, if the macular edema is allowed to persist or get worst, permanent damage can occur. With time, the entire macula can be damaged and vision can drop. Patients can become legally blind from macular edema alone.

From studies such as the ETDRS, we now know that macular edema, if it is clinically significant, should be treated with the laser. Laser surgery should be performed even if the vision is good, because fluid and substances which leak into the macula can be quite damaging. Laser surgery, when successful, can stop the progressive loss of vision, but it cannot restore vision. For example, if there is 10 percent vision loss, successful laser surgery would only be able to stop the loss at 10 percent. There would likely not be any improvement in the vision. Therefore, laser surgery should be performed before there has been any vision loss. This often is difficult to understand from the patient's perspective, because surgery is being recommended for what seems to be not a problem.

Retinal Detachment

The proliferation of new blood vessels often leads to the accumulation of blood vessels on the surface of the retina. As we discussed earlier, these new blood vessels can bleed; this condition is called a vitreous hemorrhage. With time, these new blood vessels can mature. With maturity, they become white, contract, and act like scar tissue.

Contraction of these new blood vessels can cause the retina to be lifted from its normal position and become detached. When this happens, the rods and cones stop functioning and light is not perceived. If the retinal detachment occurs in the macula, it is easy to see how vision loss can occur. Early on, detachment of the macula may be noticed as distortion in vision. With increasing detachment, there is progressive loss of vision.

The treatment for retinal detachment is repair. If the detachment occurs outside the macula, the patient may not even notice it. In these circumstances, the retinal detachment often may remain stable. The ophthalmologist may just want to closely follow these cases. However, if the detachment affects or is threatening the macula, surgery should be performed to release the traction from the contracting scar tissue. Release of these contractures will often result in less distortion and improvement in vision.

Neovascular Glaucoma

If the proliferation of new blood vessels occurs in the drainage network of the eye (trabecular meshwork), pressure can build up inside the eye. The pressure rise often can be quite abrupt. Unlike three conditions discussed above, neovascular glaucoma can be quite painful.

Neovascular glaucoma causes vision loss through high intraocular pressures. The high pressure leads to damage to the optic nerve. With a damaged optic nerve, signals from the retina cannot be communicated to the brain. Even if the retina is healthy, there is no connection to the brain. The end result is loss of vision and blindness.

Neovascular glaucoma usually requires a two-pronged attack. Laser treatment is applied to the retina to destroy the impetus for new blood vessel formation. In addition, eyedrops are prescribed to lower the pressure in the eye. If the pressure cannot be controlled by these methods, surgery may be necessary. To solve this problem, many ophthalmologists choose to create a new drain by implanting an artificial valve to relieve the pressure inside the eye.

Risk of Vision Loss

In eyes affected by diabetes, vision loss often is divided into two categories: Severe visual loss (SVL) and moderate visual loss. Severe visual loss (vision less than 20/800) is vision loss so severe that patients have trouble seeing the big "E" on the chart from 10 feet away. Legal blindness is vision less than 20/200, but patients who are legally blind can still walk around unassisted. You can be legally blind and still function well. Severe visual loss, however, usually means one is not able to get around by oneself.

Moderate visual loss can be roughly thought of as losing half of your current vision. For example, going from 20/20 to 20/40 or from 20/100 to 20/200 is said to be moderate visual loss.

What are my chances of severe visual loss?

Permanent, severe visual loss from diabetes is quite uncommon today. However, certain eyes with high-risk characteristics, such as moderate amounts of neurovascularization and vitreous hemorrhage, are more likely to develop severe visual loss. If you develop high-risk characteristics or show signs of developing them, your eye doctor will probably recommend laser treatment. If left untreated, eyes with high-risk characteristics have a 25 to 30 percent chance of severe visual loss within two years.

Table 7.1 describes the chances of developing high-risk characteristics with each level of retinopathy. The table lists the risks for eyes with nonproliferative and proliferative diabetic retinopathy. Eyes that have neovascularization (growth of new blood vessels) are considered to have proliferative diabetic retinopathy (PDR), while eyes without neovascularization have nonproliferative diabetic retinopathy (NPDR). Eyes with nonproliferative diabetic retinopathy are further divided into mild, moderate, and severe NPDR. Eyes with proliferative diabetic retinopathy are categorized as PDR with or without high-risk characteristics.

We now know from studies such as the Diabetes Control and Complications Trial (DCCT) that good blood glucose control can keep your retinopathy from progressing. With proper control of diabetes, periodic monitoring by your ophthalmologist, and laser treatment when high-risk characteristics develop, severe visual loss can be prevented.

Table 7.1   CHANCES OF DEVELOPING HIGH-RISK CHARACTERISTICS WITH VARYING LEVELS OF RETINOPATHY

Level of retinopathy	In 1 year (%)	In 3 years (%)	In 5 years (%)
Mild NPDR*	1.2	6.5	15.2
Moderate NPDR	8.1	24.7	39.2
Severe NPDR	17.1	44.4	57.8
Early PDR**	21.5	52.8	62.8

* NPDR = Nonproliferative diabetic retinopathy (retinopathy without neovascularization).
** PDR = Proliferative diabetic retinopathy (retinopathy with neovascularization).

What are my chances of getting some vision back after suffering severe visual loss?

Visual loss is best prevented with good blood glucose control and timely laser treatment. However, once severe visual loss develops, only about 30 percent of patients will have improved vision after treatment. Vision of 20/40 or better is required for driving in most states, but less than 20 percent will return to this level of vision, and less than 30 percent will have improvement better than 20/100.

Those that lose vision from vitreous hemorrhage and macular edema are more likely to regain vision with treatment. The good news is that most people have two eyes. Only a small proportion of people have severe visual loss in both eyes. Even if vision is lost in one eye, vision may still be good in the other one.

What are my chances of moderate visual loss?

Moderate visual loss is much more common. Moderate visual loss often develops in eyes with macular edema. If clinically significant macular edema is present (CSME), the chance of developing moderate visual loss in two years is somewhere around 10 to 20 percent. If laser treatment is promptly applied to fix the leaky areas causing the macular edema, the risk of visual loss can be reduced by half.

Preventing Visual Loss

Although diabetes mellitus is the leading cause of vision loss in working-age Americans, many patients have diabetes without developing significant visual loss. Preventing vision loss includes good serum glucose control and keeping appointments with your eye doctor.

Good glucose control means different things for Type I and Type II diabetes. For patients with Type I diabetes, good control means frequent monitoring of blood sugar and adjustment of insulin dose. For older patients with Type II diabetes, good control means weight loss, exercise, and a diet low in fat and sugars with plenty of fruits and vegetables.

Appointments with your ophthalmologist are also very important. Upon examining your eyes, your ophthalmologist can evaluate the level of retinopathy, determine the prognosis of your eyes, and decide whether any treatment is necessary.

8

Vitamins and Eye Disease

Americans favor new ideas and like to follow trends. Sometimes, scientific knowledge and research develops that support a new idea. This new idea becomes accepted, standard teaching. At other times, however, ideas are merely fads, not supported by scientific investigation. As more research disproves the idea, the fad falls from favor.

In recent years, many people have become interested in vitamins and their role in health. The interest has arisen because most people live hectic lives and do not eat a healthy diet. Instead of improving their diets, people hope that taking vitamin pills will be a "quick fix." Even with fast-food consumption in the United States, vitamin deficiencies are still quite rare. Even so, they are blamed for many problems. Newspapers and magazines are full of impressive claims of diseases cured with vitamins. However, most of the claims are not supported by sound scientific evidence.

Vitamins are substances that are essential for the normal functioning of the body (metabolism) that are not made by the body and must be supplied by an outside source, such as in the diet. Recommended daily allowances are known for most vitamins. (See Table 8.1.) However, the ideal or optimal amount of vitamin intake is not known. In fact, the amount probably varies from person to person. While poor eating habits and some ethnic dietary customs may result in poor nutrition and inadequate vitamin intake, it is difficult to avoid vitamins in the diet.

Minerals are involved in many bodily functions. Copper and iron are necessary for blood building. Sodium, chloride, and potassium maintain the electrical balance in the blood and cells for the function of the nerves and muscles. Manganese and other trace elements are widely found in foods, and almost no one needs to take supplemental amounts. Some experts suggest calcium supplementation to prevent osteoporosis. Iron supplementation may be helpful for people with certain kinds of anemias, for young women, and for patients with renal failure. Sometimes it is necessary to avoid certain minerals. People with hypertension should avoid sodium. In patients with kidney failure, potassium may build up and put the heart rhythm at risk. In these cases, potassium has to be restricted.

The critical role of vitamin A in vision is well recognized. Deficiencies in this nutrient, still common in the developing world, are associated with night blindness in the early stages that can progress to perforation of the eye and blindness in the late stages. Deficiencies of B_6 and B_{12} have been associated with nerve damage (neuropathy), but true deficiencies are really rare. Again, these conditions are

Table 8.1 VITAMINS, FUNCTIONS, AND BEST FOOD SOURCES

Vitamin	Best Sources	Functions	Deficiency Symptoms
A Retinol Carotene	Liver, eggs, dark green and deep orange fruits and vegetables, dairy products	Growth and repair of body tissues, infection resistance, bone and tooth formation, necessary for night vision	Night blindness, drying of the eyes, rough skin, impaired bone growth
B₁ Thiamine	Wheat germ, liver, pork, whole grains, enriched grains, dried beans	Carbohydrate metabolism, appetite maintenance, nerve function, growth, muscle tone	Mental confusion, muscle weakness, edema, fatigue, loss of appetite
B₂ Riboflavin	Dairy products, green leafy vegetables, whole grains, enriched grains	Necessary for fat, carbohydrate, and protein metabolism, cell respiration, formation of antibodies and red blood cells	Sensitivity of eyes to light, cracks in corners of the mouth, dermatitis around nose and lips
B₆	Fish, poultry, lean meats, whole grains	Necessary for fat, carbohydrate, and protein metabolism	Dermatitis, anemia, nausea, smooth tongue

continued

Table 8.1 *continued*

Vitamin	Best Sources	Functions	Deficiency Symptoms
B₁₂ Cobalamin	Organ meats, lean meat, fish, poultry, eggs, dairy products	Carbohydrate, fat, and protein metabolism, maintains health of nervous system, blood cell formation	Pernicious anemia, numbness and tingling in fingers and toes
Biotin	Egg yolks, organ meats, dark green vegetables; also made by microorganisms in the intestinal tract	Carbohydrate, fat, and protein metabolism, formation of fatty acids, helps utilize B vitamins	Not seen under normal circumstances; pale, dry scaly skin, depression, poor appetite
Folic Acid	Green leafy vegetables, organ meats, dried beans	Red blood cell formation, protein metabolism, cell division	Anemia, diarrhea, smooth tongue, poor growth
Niacin	Meat, poultry, fish, nuts, whole grains, enriched grains, dried beans	Fat, carbohydrate, and protein metabolism, health of skin, tongue, and digestive system, blood circulation	General fatigue, digestive disorders, irritability, loss of appetite, skin disorders

Vitamin	Sources	Function	Deficiency Symptoms
Pantothenic Acid	Lean meats, whole grains, legumes	Converts nutrients into energy, formation of some fats, vitamin utilization	Not seen under normal circumstances; vomiting, severe abdominal cramps, fatigue, tingling hands and feet
C, Ascorbic Acid	Citrus fruits, melon, berries, vegetables	Helps heal wounds, strengthens blood vessels, collagen maintenance, resistance to infection	Bleeding gums, slow-healing wounds, bruising, aching joints, nosebleeds, anemia
D, Calciferol	Egg yolks, organ meats, fortified milk; also made in skin exposed to sunlight	Bone and teeth formation	Poor bone growth, rickets, osteomalacia, muscle twitching
E, Tocopherol	Vegetable oils, margarine, wheat germ, nuts, dark green vegetables, whole grains	Maintains cell membranes, protects vitamin A and essential fatty acids from oxidation, red blood cell formation	Not seen in humans except after prolonged impairment of fat absorption; neurological abnormalities
K	Green leafy vegetables, fruits, cereals, dairy products	Important in formation of blood clotting agents	Tendency to hemorrhage

extremely unusual in the United States. A major research interest for vitamins and minerals is whether they provide protection from oxidative damage in various disease states, particularly eye disease. Many people believe that taking antioxidant supplements will prevent vision loss from oxidative damage. Currently, the role of vitamin C, E, and beta carotene antioxidants in the prevention of cataract and age-related macular degeneration is under scientific investigation.

In this chapter, we will discuss oxidative damage, antioxidants, and the role of antioxidant supplementation.

What is oxidative damage?

Chemical reactions occur every moment of our lives. They are an essential part of metabolism. However, there are certain chemical reactions that can cause injury to the eye if they occur in areas that are sensitive to damage. Oxidation is one chemical reaction that may be damaging to certain parts of the eye, such as the lens and retina. Oxidation is essential to their function, but too much oxidation is damaging. Excess oxidation may occur when highly reactive chemical substances, such as free radicals, are present. Free radicals occur both naturally (produced by the cell's metabolism) and through exposure to light (see Figure 8.1). Examples of free radicals include singlet oxygen, superoxide, and hydrogen peroxide. Because free radicals are normally present in the body, the body has ways of protecting itself against oxidative damage. In areas of normal oxidation activity, the body maintains reserves of antioxidants that can quench excess oxidation reactions that "get out of hand." Antioxidants include vitamins C and E

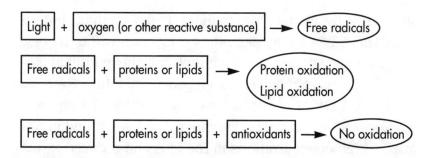

Figure 8.1 **Free radicals**

and beta carotene. In addition, the body maintains certain enzymes that break down free radicals when too many accumulate.

Some scientists have hypothesized that taking antioxidant supplements may prevent cataract and retinal diseases by preventing the oxidation of proteins and fats in the lens and retina. Following the same line of thinking, others have suggested taking minerals that are part of the enzymes that break down free radicals.

Antioxidants

Vitamin C
Vitamin C has an important function in the body. A lack of this vitamin causes scurvy, the disease of sailors in earlier days. English sailors who took lime juice to prevent scurvy on long voyages were known as "limeys." Vitamin C is found in citrus fruits and juices, cantaloupes, strawberries, raw cabbage, and green peppers.

There has been controversy about taking massive doses of vitamin C to prevent the common cold. This theory was suggested by Nobel Prize winner Linus Pauling, but to date, there has been no evidence to confirm his theory. Other people suggest that vitamin C may be helpful in diabetes, but this also has not been proven helpful.

Application of the antioxidant properties of vitamin C has focused on cataracts. Vitamin C has been found in relatively high concentrations in the lens and reduced levels have been found in cataractous lenses. Taking oral supplements can raise the level of vitamin C in the lens.

Vitamin E

Vitamin E (tocopherol) is a fat-soluble antioxidant. In addition to preventing oxidation reactions from "running amok," tocopherol also helps maintain the integrity of cell membranes in the lens. Tocopherol has been found to reduce lens damage in rabbits and to prevent cataracts in laboratory rats. While vitamin E is found in the human lens, it is not known whether supplementation increases its level in the lens.

Carotenoids

Beta carotene is probably the best-known antioxidant. It is a vegetable precursor of vitamin A and is a very effective antioxidant. Unfortunately, it is not found in high concentrations in the retina. While the antioxidant activity of beta carotene is well established, other carotenoids, such as lycopene and lutein, are also effective antioxidants and present in higher concentrations inside the retina.

Riboflavin

Riboflavin is required for the body's synthesis of flavin adenine dinucleotide (FAD), a cofactor for the antioxidant enzyme glutathione reductase. In several animal studies, a deficiency of riboflavin resulted in cataract formation.

Selenium

Selenium is a constituent of glutathione peroxidase, an enzyme whose primary metabolic role is destruction of free radicals such as hydrogen peroxide. Gluthathione peroxidase is present in the retina and the retinal pigment epithelium.

Manganese

Manganese is an essential part of the superoxide dismutase, another enzyme that destroys free radicals.

Zinc

Zinc occurs in ocular tissues in high concentrations, particularly in the retinal pigment epithelial layer of the retina. Deficiency of this nutrient may lead to night blindness and impaired dark adaptation. A role for zinc deficiency in retinal degeneration has also been proposed.

Cataract

As we discussed in Chapter 2, a cataract is a lens that has undergone changes that lead to the reduction in the clarity of the lens. This loss of clarity is due to changes in the proteins of the lens. With time and age, proteins degenerate and form opaque substances. Many scientists believe that this degeneration process is due to oxidation. These same scientists believe that antioxidants may help prevent cataracts by preventing the formation of the opaque proteins.

As mentioned, vitamin C has been found in relatively high concentrations in the lens; reduced levels have been found in the cataractous lens. Laboratory experiments have shown that vitamin C can prevent cataract formation in rats exposed to strong light. Whether this applies to humans is not known. Some studies have shown that people with cataracts have lower blood levels of vitamin C. However, other studies have not found such an association. We do know that vitamin C taken by mouth can get into the lens. In one experiment, patients who took vitamin C immediately before cataract surgery had higher levels of vitamin C in their cataracts, compared to those patients who did not take vitamin C.

There is some evidence that vitamin E may prevent certain types of cataract. However, most studies in humans have not confirmed a link between dietary vitamin E intake and cataract formation.

There are no published animal studies that investigate whether carotenoids have any relation to cataract. There have been several human studies on this relationship, however. Most of these studies have shown that dietary intake of carotenoids was associated with a lower risk of cataract. In one study, the Nurse's Health Study, the carotenoid intake was correlated with foods. Interestingly, the food with the greatest source of beta carotene, carrots, was not shown to protect against cataracts.

Animal studies have not been conclusive about the role of riboflavin and cataract formation. Some human studies have shown a decrease in cataract formation with higher levels of riboflavin, but the reduction in risk has been small.

Age-Related Macular Degeneration

Age-related macular degeneration (AMD) is the leading cause of irreversible blindness among older Americans. As many as 15 million people older than fifty years may have this disease. There is very little known about the cause of AMD. Many scientists believe that light and light-induced oxidation of the retina are important factors leading to it.

As we discussed earlier in this chapter, light leads to the formation of free radicals. These free radicals then oxidize and destroy proteins and lipids. One area of the eye with a large accumulation of lipids is the retina. In fact, the light-sensitive portion of the retina, called the rods and cones layer, is entirely lipid.

Laboratory experiments have shown that animals deprived of vitamins C and E tend to develop a condition very similar to AMD. Vitamin E is a fat-soluble antioxidant that can protect the lipids in the retina from oxidative destruction by interrupting free radical reactions. Vitamin E has also been theorized to protect against the eye damage that occurs in human infants who are born prematurely (retinopathy of prematurity). However, there is little human evidence that vitamin C or E provides protection against AMD.

Few studies have examined the relationship between the important minerals and AMD in humans. In one very small study, oral zinc supplementation was associated with a lower chance of developing end-stage AMD. However, this study is controversial because the placebo group had an unusually high rate of disease.

The Eye Disease Case Control Study was a study done

at several large universities and private practices. This study found that the risk of advanced AMD was related to the level of carotenoids in the blood. It measured the levels of several antioxidants in patients with advanced AMD and other patients without AMD. The patients with AMD tended to have lower levels of antioxidants in their blood.

To investigate the association between blood levels of these nutrients and dietary intake, patients were asked to fill out a questionnaire about their diets. Using complicated analyses, the study showed that the main carotenoid protective against AMD is not beta carotene, the carotenoid found in carrots, but lutein, the carotenoid found in spinach, collard greens, and other green leafy vegetables.

Diabetic Retinopathy

At present, there is no evidence that antioxidants affect the course of diabetic retinopathy. Persons with or without diabetes who eat a well-planned diet do not require vitamin supplements. Many people take multivitamin supplements because they rely on fast foods or because they do not like fruits and vegetables. These supplements are probably harmless, but they do not replace the nutrients found in a balanced diet.

Vitamin Supplement Use

Vitamin preparations have a sales volume of over 4 billion dollars a year in the United States. Many are harmless, because excess vitamins are destroyed or eliminated from the body. However, some vitamins can be harmful in very large doses. There are two types of vitamins: water-soluble vitamins, such as vitamins B and C, and fat-soluble vitamins, such as A, D, K, and E. When large doses of water soluble vitamins are consumed, most of the excess is not absorbed but is lost in the urine. In extremely high doses, they can be stored in the liver and cause toxicity. High doses of fat-soluble vitamins are deposited in the body's fat and are harmful. High doses of vitamin A can be damaging to pregnant women and their fetuses. High doses of vitamin A harm the central nervous system and may cause birth defects. Vitamin D also should be used with caution. Children can have toxic reactions with 50,000 IU daily. High doses can lead to calcium deposits (calcification) in the eyes and other parts of the body. Other possible effects include convulsions, acute pancreatitis, elevations of triglycerides, nausea, diarrhea, blurred vision, headache, and bone loss.

Taking high doses of antioxidants has been shown in one study to actually increase the risk of death for smokers. In 1994, the ATBC Trial (Alpha-Tocopherol Beta Carotene Cancer Prevention Study) reported its results. This was a study that enrolled 29,133 male smokers from Finland between the ages of fifty and sixty-nine. These patients were randomly assigned to get either alpha-tocopherol (50 mg/day), beta carotene (20 mg/day), both supplements, or placebo. The patients in this study were followed for five to eight years and had 99 percent compliance. Contrary to what everyone expected, there was a higher risk of death and lung cancer in those given beta carotene. This was a very surprising finding. A lot of scientists believed that this finding was just chance and discounted these results. In 1996, the CARET Study (beta-CArotene Retinol

Efficacy Trial) studied 18,314 workers treated with beta carotene and placebo and came to the same conclusion. In yet another study, the Physician Health Study, beta carotene was found to be ineffective in preventing other cancers or heart disease. So far, beta carotene has not been found to be effective for any disease studied. For certain problems, beta carotene may even be harmful.

There has been much talk about supplementing zinc to prevent macular degeneration. Zinc may be less harmful than beta carotene, but high dietary consumption of zinc may lead to anemia and a reduction in blood levels of the "good cholesterol," HDL (high density lipoprotein).

Summary

The decision to take vitamins should be based on need, safety, and cost. Persons with or without diabetes who consume a well-planned diet do not require vitamin supplements. At present, there is no sound scientific evidence that taking vitamin supplements will prevent eye disease. In certain circumstances, some dietary supplements may even be harmful. Smokers probably should avoid taking beta carotene supplements. A better preventive measure is eating a well-balanced diet low in fats and sweets and including at least five servings of fruits and vegetables a day.

9

Pregnancy and Diabetic Eye Disease

In the past, pregnancy in women with diabetes posed significant risks to both mother and child. Today, pregnancy is much safer. However, special care is still required and successful outcomes cannot always be expected. To be sure that both mother and child receive optimum care, pregnancy in a diabetic woman should be carefully scripted. There should be planning and preparation well before conception.

Women planning conception must understand the risks pregnancy poses to their own health and to the developing child. To adequately consider these issues, medical care of the diabetic mother should involve an obstetrician who is skilled in the management of high-risk cases and a neonatologist (a pediatrician who specializes in care of newborns). Maternal deaths now rarely occur, and infant survival in experienced centers is almost 98 percent.

In addition to risks to maternal health, diabetes leads to increased risks of birth defects. Defects can affect the heart, brain, and bones and muscles. With proper diabetes control during pregnancy, however, the risk of these defects can be reduced. Good blood glucose control during the first twelve weeks is most critical for lowering the number of major birth defects.

Pregnancy and Diabetes

One important difference between pregnancy in women with and without diabetes is the increased risk of developing ketoacidosis in diabetics. Pregnancy, with its fluctuating hormone levels, predisposes the diabetic woman to a much more rapid onset of severe ketoacidosis. This occurs because pregnant women require more insulin than nonpregnant women. In women without diabetes, the pancreas can respond and produce enough insulin for this additional demand.

Even in some women without a prior history of diabetes, high blood glucose levels may be observed during pregnancy. This occurs because the pancreas which normally produces enough insulin, is not able to keep up with the increasing demands of pregnancy. This condition is called gestational diabetes. Women who require insulin before pregnancy will usually require one to three times as much during their pregnancy.

Gestational Diabetes

High blood glucose levels are found in 1 to 2 percent of all pregnant women. Of patients with high blood sugars during pregnancy, only 10 percent were known to have diabetes before conceiving. Gestational diabetes is more likely to occur in women with other diabetic family members, among women who are overweight, and among those over the age of thirty. A previous pregnancy with complications suggestive of maternal diabetes is associated with an increased risk of developing diabetes during the current pregnancy. Possible complications are macrosomia, or a large baby, and miscarriages. If you have any risk factors, your doctor may want to test your ability to deal with glucose (glucose tolerance test). In this test, you will be asked to drink a beverage with a known amount of sugar. Over the next couple of hours, the sugar level in your blood will be measured. Your ability to handle the sugar load will determine whether you have diabetes.

Because proper blood sugar levels reduce the likelihood of diabetic complications in the fetus, even mild forms of gestational diabetes are treated. The good news is that even if insulin is used during the pregnancy, it may not be required after delivery. In addition, gestational diabetes usually does not lead to any permanent visual change. Pregnant women often notice some blurriness in their vision. This blurriness likely arises from lens swelling caused by the high blood sugars and is usually transient.

Effects of Pregnancy on Diabetes

The insulin doses and food required to control diabetes will change during pregnancy, but after the delivery, the treatment program becomes similar to that previously used. The overall health of the mother usually returns to her prepregnant state. Any increase in risks of complications, such as worsening of diabetic retinopathy, often slows or stops progressing after delivery. However, a few conditions require special attention because even temporary worsening may be dangerous.

Glucose Control During Pregnancy

As always, the aim of diabetes treatment is to maintain good blood glucose control, and keep blood glucose levels as close to normal as possible. The goal of treatment is a fasting capillary (finger-stick) blood glucose level of 60 to 100 mg percent and a level of 100 to 150 mg percent two hours after eating. To achieve this, it may be necessary to test the blood at home at least four times daily: fasting (before breakfast), and two hours after breakfast, lunch, and dinner.

Diet

During pregnancy, as with all diabetes treatment, the importance of diet cannot be overemphasized. In addition, the diet must contain more calories, including increased carbohydrates and protein to provide for the needs of both mother and fetus. The balance of insulin, food, and activity may need many readjustments during pregnancy!

Eye Findings During Pregnancy

In general, pregnancy tends to increase the progression of retinopathy. For example, eyes that have severe nonproliferative or early proliferative diabetic retinopathy might rapidly progress to high-risk characteristics. Eyes that may only require close follow-up during the nonpregnant state might require laser treatment during pregnancy. Because pregnancy may speed up the eye changes of diabetes and because these changes can result in permanent vision loss, conception should be postponed until these problems are treated. Eyes with macular edema and eyes with proliferative retinopathy or severe nonproliferative diabetic retinopathy may need laser treatment and be allowed to stabilize before pregnancy.

Because it is so important to know the baseline condition of the retina, the woman with diabetes who is considering pregnancy should see an ophthalmologist before conception. The ophthalmologist can assess any retinopathy and whether laser treatment is needed to avoid progressive damage from the pregnancy. After conception, an eye exam should be performed during the first trimester. At that time, your eye doctor can further assess how your retinopathy is progressing. Should the retinopathy be increasing, additional follow-up and treatment may be necessary. There is no effect on the unborn baby if laser treatment is required during pregnancy.

Delivery

Babies born to women with diabetes tend to be bigger and have higher birth weights than average. Diabetic mothers have a higher risk of miscarriages and stillbirths. Because early delivery is thought to reduce the risk to the fetus during the later weeks of pregnancy, delivery used to be induced earlier in women with diabetes. Babies sometimes were delivered as early as four to six weeks before their due dates. With modern care and monitoring, the risk has been reduced so that delivery is now performed between the thirty-sixth and thirty-eighth weeks. By the thirty-eighth week most babies are mature enough to deliver, but delivery sometimes can be delayed until term (forty weeks).

Infants of diabetic mothers traditionally have been larger than those born to women without diabetes. This large size is called macrosomia, and it carries with it health problems for the child, including an increased need for a cesarean delivery and a greater chance of birth trauma. Cesarean deliveries are needed in about 20 to 30 percent of all pregnant women with diabetes, although their necessity is controversial.

Cesarean section may also be recommended for certain women who are at a high risk of vitreous hemorrhage. The bearing down that is required during delivery may increase pressure on the eye vessels, which may cause them to rupture. As we discussed in Chapters 6 and 8, vitreous hemorrhage can cause visual loss. However, the visual loss can be transient. Even if the vitreous hemorrhage persists and causes prolonged visual loss, vitrectomy surgery can be performed to remove the blood and clear the vision. The type of birth best for you and your baby, a cesarian or vaginal delivery, should be based on a discussion among your obstetrician, neonatologist, and ophthalmologist.

Effect on Fetal Eye Development

The most common eye birth defect associated with maternal diabetes is optic nerve hypoplasia, although the frequency is probably less than 1 percent. The optic nerve is the part of the eye that connects the eye to the brain. It provides the conduit by which light signals from the retina are conveyed to the brain for perception. Optic nerve hypoplasia means a small optic nerve. Fortunately, many children with optic nerve hypoplasia do not have significant vision loss.

Conclusion

Intensive monitoring by a health care team of the mother before conception, throughout pregnancy, and during delivery has reduced the risk to maternal health. Vision loss from pregnancy-induced progression of retinopathy is still a concern. Good glucose control, in addition to vigilant monitoring by an ophthalmologist, can reduce the risk of vision loss. Uncontrolled diabetes can cause birth defects. Fortunately, its most common birth defect, optic nerve hypoplasia, is rare and is often not associated with significant visual loss.

If you are considering pregnancy, be certain to see your diabetologist, obstetrician, and ophthalmologist before you conceive.

10

Childhood Diabetes and the Eye

Y ou have recently learned that your child has insulin dependent diabetes (IDDM), also called Type I diabetes. For a parent or relative, learning that his or her child has diabetes can come as a total shock, throwing the whole world into chaos. You are probably reading this chapter because you want to do whatever it takes to protect your child's life and health. This includes ensuring that your child sees well.

The more you learn about diabetes and how it works, the better you will be able to help your child live with it. Diabetes will not prevent you or your child from leading a full and active life, but diabetes does make it tougher. However, the risk of blindness from diabetes in the teenage and adolescent years is very low. Teaching your child the importance of having his or her eyes examined can give him or her a head start in preventing complications later in life.

Chapter Ten

What is insulin dependent diabetes?

As your pediatrician may have explained, the pancreas is an organ located beneath the stomach which makes insulin, a hormone. Insulin allows your child's body to use glucose, a form of sugar produced when starches are digested for energy. Hormones are molecules which are secreted by one organ and cause another organ to have an effect. For example, the sun, when it shines, causes the flowers to grow and blossom. Insulin is necessary to remove glucose from the bloodstream and move it into the body's cells, which need the fuel to function. The amount of insulin required depends on how active your child is (the amount of fuel he or she needs) and how many calories are eaten. Stress and illness can also throw off the normal balance of insulin, diet, and activity. As a general rule, insulin and exercise decrease the blood level of glucose; eating increases the level of blood glucose. Elevated blood glucose is called hyperglycemia (*hyper*—too much, *glyc*—glucose, *emia*—in the blood). Hypoglycemia is the exact opposite, too little glucose in the blood.

Your child takes insulin to control the diabetes, but insulin is not a cure. Insulin cannot prevent the complications of diabetes. While insulin can control the diabetes, there are still serious complications which can develop later in life. These complications include nephropathy (kidney failure), neuropathy (nerve damage), and retinopathy (retina or vision loss).

The Diabetes Control and Complications Trial (DCCT) showed that when blood sugar was maintained at a normal level, or below 150, through intensified treatment, the complications of diabetes were reduced. Tight control requires a commitment to check the glucose level at least four times daily and adjust the insulin as well as to work closely with a qualified diabetes health care team. It entails a huge commitment. However, the trial found that low sugar, or hypoglycemia, occurred three times more frequently in the intensified treatment group. It concluded that intensive treatment was not for everyone, especially young children. You should understand the results of the DCCT and discuss with your pediatrician the best diabetes management approach for your child or adolescent.

Is anyone else in my family at risk for diabetes mellitus?

If your child has Type I diabetes and a parent also has Type II, there is an increased risk of Type I diabetes in other children in the family.

How do the results of the DCCT apply to my child?

In general, the DCCT studied Type I diabetics between the ages of thirteen and thirty-nine years. Approximately 14 percent of participants were thirteen to eighteen years old. Participants were assigned to either of two treatment groups; the first group was the standard or conventional treatment group, and the second was the intensified treatment group.

The standard treatment involved checking the blood sugar once or twice daily and administering insulin. The intensified treatment regimen involved self-monitoring a minimum of four times daily, with administration of insulin by multiple injections or with a continuous insulin infusion pump. This intensified treatment was structured within an environment of diabetes professionals that included diabetologists (physicians specializing in diabetes), diabetes nurse educators, behavioral scientists, nutritionists, and social workers.

The results conclusively showed that the intensified treatment group obtained lower glucose levels, lower serum hemoglobin A_{1c}, and had less complications; however, the rate of severe hypoglycemia was three times higher in the intensive treatment group than in the standard treatment group. Children under age thirteen were not included in this study because of their continuing brain development and lack of both physical and psychological maturation.

Hypoglycemia is a serious threat when one attempts strict metabolic control and may affect the development of the brain in the most formative developmental years and can lead to seizures and coma. Children and preadolescents frequently have erratic blood sugars with standard treatment because of their inconsistent diets and bursts of unpredictable activity. It is possible that the threefold risk of severe hypoglycemia associated with the intensive treatment group could have a more devastating effect on brain development and intellectual function in younger children.

It should be emphasized that the adolescents who participated in the DCCT were self-motivated and were not participating at the sole request of their parents. The type of personal involvement required for intensive treatment is not a personality trait common to children under age thirteen. Don't take it personally if your pediatrician doesn't recommend intensive therapy for your child!

These findings do not mean that HbA_{1c} levels above normal are desirable for children. Normal blood glucose is still desirable for Type I children of all ages, so long as it does not cause severe hypoglycemia or emotional problems for the child and the family. The goal should be to implement strategies that avoid hypoglycemia rather than promote hyperglycemia.

The DCCT study recommended tight control in Type I diabetes. Does this apply to my child as well?

Tight control should not be attempted in anyone unable or unwilling to participate actively in their own glucose control management. Therefore, tight control should not be used in infants less than age two. In children between the ages of two and seven, extreme caution should be used in adopting tight control because of the risk of hypoglycemic episodes. Because the DCCT studied Type I patients over age thirteen, some diabetes doctors do not advocate a regimen of tight control in anyone less than thirteen years of age. Many behavioral scientists do not think that children younger than age thirteen can be self-motivated enough to comply with all the work necessary to practice tight control. Despite a parent's best wishes for tight control, the child or adolescent must be an active and willing participant.

Hypoglycemia can impair normal brain development, and as mentioned, it can occur more commonly in children because food intake, activity levels, and adherence to treatment schedules are more unpredictable.

Parents whose children have experienced a hypoglycemic episode are more likely to fear another one and adjust their children's sugar to run higher. Fear of hypoglycemia should be discussed with a diabetes educator, pediatrician, or family physician. Adolescents who experience a severe hypoglycemic episode are more likely to report fear of another episode, generally worry, and perceive negatively the effect of diabetes on their daily lives.

In preadolescents, microvascular, or small vessel complications were rare. The need for tight control may be less important than in postpubertal patients.

Do I need to take my child to a "diabetes specialist," since the DCCT included diabetes specialists in their study?

It is estimated that less than 5 percent of all diabetic patients in the United States receive care from a diabetes specialist. A somewhat higher number, 20 percent of all children and adolescents with Type I diabetes, receive therapeutic guidance from a university-based or diabetes specialty center where the therapeutic team is an integral component of management.

Today, few primary care physicians receive specialized training about current diabetes management, and few of these physicians or their patients have access to the multiple benefits of a diabetes therapeutic team. Medicine has a long way to go in the transition to the coordinated diabetes management team. Managed care companies must recognize the importance of management teams and place value on the nonphysician teammates who include social workers, psychologists, diabetic educators, and nutritionists. They must likewise recognize the advantages of preventive care and careful screening as well as frequent visits.

What is diabetic retinopathy?

Retinopathy means there is damage to the retina, the lining of the inside of the eye. The eye is very similar in its design to a camera. The retina is like the film portion of the camera. The lens inside the eye and the glasses which are worn by some people function like the lens on the camera body.

Retinopathy is a result of long-standing, chronic disease. Changes in the retina take years to occur, and these changes usually follow puberty or the growth spurt if they are going to take place. In the DCCT, the results showed that it takes approximately three years of lowered HbA_{1c} levels before the benefits of less complications become apparent.

Retinopathy is of two types: nonproliferative and proliferative. The nonproliferative type is less advanced and means that the blood vessels are not normal and the retina is mildly sick. There may be dot and blot hemorrhages in the retina, tiny aneurysms or ballooning out of the blood vessels, and areas of cotton wool spots which will signify to the ophthalmologist that diabetic changes are taking place.

Is diabetic retinopathy preventable?

The importance of education and prevention cannot be overemphasized. Despite our ability to treat patients who develop proliferative retinopathy with lasers to prevent blindness, we still see young people in their twentiess and thirties who were unaware of the importance of eye examinations and who present with severe retinopathy that could have been diagnosed earlier with proper referral and screening. Multiple studies have conclusively shown that treating proliferative disease with laser can reduce the risk of severe vision loss by 50 percent.

One should not relax vigilance just because the prepubertal years are relatively free of complications; these years are important in the evolution of the tissue damage which may become apparent in adolescence and young adulthood.

What are the current guidelines for pediatric diabetic eye examinations?

The American Academy of Pediatrics and the American Academy of Ophthalmology are currently studying screening recommendations for diabetic retinopathy in children with Type I diabetes. The American Academy of Ophthalmology and the American Diabetes Association suggest that children with Type I diabetes should have an eye examination five years after the onset of the disease and every year thereafter. They want to ensure that your child is starting off with the best visual potential in both eyes. This initial visit is meant to educate the pediatric patient and his or her family about diabetic retinopathy, screen for any early disease, and provide an opportunity to familiarize the family with the ophthalmologist who will care for the child, ask questions to alleviate concerns, and impart at an early age to the child the importance of routine eye examinations.

The examination schedule in Table 10.1 is suggested for the child (birth to twenty years) with Type I diabetes who is asymptomatic (without known eye findings).

Who should perform eye examinations?

Studies suggest that an ophthalmologist, who is a medical doctor, is more likely to detect the changes of diabetic

Table 10.1   SUGGESTED OPHTHALMOLOGIC EXAMINATION SCHEDULE
FOR ASYMPTOMATIC CHILDREN WITH TYPE I DIABETES

Examination	Frequency
Initial discussion	Within the first year after diagnosis, child and/or parents should receive counseling by a pediatrician, pediatric endocrinologist, or ophthalmologist regarding the need for ophthalmic examination and early intervention
Initial examination*	Prepubertal—examination at nine years of age if diabetes duration is less than three years Onset at puberty—examination three years post diagnosis
Follow-up examination*	Annually
During pregnancy*	During first trimester, then every three months until delivery

*Abnormal findings may necessitate more frequent follow-up examinations.

retinopathy than other eye care practitioners. Ophthalmologists are specialists trained to recognize all diseases of the eye and to treat these diseases both medically and surgically if necessary. They are trained in all subspecialties of the eye including pediatrics, glaucoma, retina, neuro-ophthalmology, and cornea/refractive surgery. They also prescribe glasses. An ophthalmologist has attended medical school and spent time training as an internist, pediatrician, or general surgeon, oftentimes managing patients with diabetes and their complications. A retina specialist is an ophthalmologist with a focus on the retina, including diabetic retinopathy.

An optometrist is also trained to recognize diseases of

the eye and to prescribe and dispense glasses. Optometrists have not gone to medical school and have spent less time training than ophthalmologists. In some states, optometrists can dispense medications. Because they have not gone to medical school, most states prohibit optometrists from dispensing medications or performing surgery of any type. An optician is a person who specializes in making glasses and fitting them.

Both ophthalmologists and optometrists are eye care specialists who wish to educate and prevent the harmful effects of diabetes in your child. If you see an optometrist for eye care, he or she may decide to refer you to an ophthalmologist or retina specialist if retinopathy is progressing or for a second opinion.

If you do not have an eye care provider, you can ask your pediatrician or contact the Juvenile Diabetes Foundation or the American Academy of Ophthalmology in your state for a referral (see Appendices).

Do I have to wait until my child can read before he or she has an eye examination?

No, your eye doctor is trained to use other methods to check vision. No age is considered too young or too old to have an eye examination.

What should I expect at my child's eye examination?

You should expect that your child will have a complete eye examination and that it will be done in such a way that your child is comfortable. Most children are relieved to discover that they won't get a shot at the eye doctor.

The examination will include sensory testing, vision testing, possibly cycloplegic refraction, slit lamp examination, and dilated examination to look at the lens, vitreous, and retina, and if your child is old enough, applanation tonometry to check the eye pressure inside the eye. This last examination is the glaucoma test. If your child cannot read or does not know letters, the ophthalmologist will use other methods of measuring vision.

In children, sensory testing is usually performed before the vision is tested. Despite its name, sensory testing does not test smell or hearing. Sensory testing checks how well the two eyes work together; it includes a test of depth perception. Your child may be asked to wear special glasses. A stereoacuity book tests depth perception and will have a fly, animals, and circles. The child may be asked to pick up the wings of the fly and point to the animals and circles which jump out of the page. Children who are not old enough to perform the test may be tested anyway so that they get used to the routine. Don't be alarmed if your child is too young to understand the test. Another test, called the Worth-4-dot, requires your child to wear a pair of red-green, round glasses. Your child will be shown a flashlight with colored spots at both a close-up range and a distant range. He or she will be asked to count the colored spots. If children can't yet count, they will be asked to touch the spots. Children usually find both tests fun.

In the infant, teller acuity cards, or grating cards can be used to evaluate vision. These cards have solid black lines which run parallel to each other and are positioned on one side of a rectangular card. The examiner cannot see on which side of the card the lines are located. There is a small central hole in the center of the card, a peephole, through which the examiner can watch the direction your infant looks. Your child will likely look at the bold black lines. The finer the black lines, the more vision your child must have in order to distinguish these lines.

In preschool children, vision can also be measured either with the E game or the picture game. The child is asked to point in the direction of the legs of the E. For example, for a regular E the child would point to the right. Another means of testing the vision is the picture game. Children may be shown pictures and asked to identify them; they may include a car, telephone, cat, or bird. Older children can often read the standard Snellen chart with all the letters of the alphabet mixed up. Don't be upset if your child misses an occasional letter on a line. Try to encourage your child to guess and encourage the shy child to do his or her best. Remember, these tests are simply a means of measuring a baseline for your unique child.

No part of the eye examination is painful. The eyedrops will often burn, but this mild effect lasts only a few seconds and is quickly forgotten.

The drops placed in your child's eyes cause dilation of the pupil in the center of the colored part of the eye, the iris. This dilation is a very important part of the diabetic child's examination. It allows the doctor to use special lenses to visualize the retina and determine the health of the eye. The lights used to perform this examination can be very bright and may cause your child's eyes to tear. Again, this tearing is a natural response and does not hurt.

Your eye doctor may want to perform a refraction to check whether your child needs glasses. A refraction will be performed at the discretion of your eye doctor based on the age of your child and his or her symptoms. If a refraction is performed in a child less than nine years old, it should be a cycloplegic refraction. For older children, this may also be advisable based on the child's symptoms.

A cycloplegic refraction uses special dilating drops. There are two basic kinds of dilating drops: those that merely make the pupil larger and those which temporarily paralyze the muscles of accommodation. The muscles of accommodation cause the natural lenses inside our eyes to change shape so that we can read up close without difficulty. As we approach the age of forty, many people begin to lose this ability to accommodate. It is this loss that leads us to the eye doctor for bifocals or makes stubborn individuals hold the paper at arm's length.

In children, these muscles of accommodation can work overtime, making it difficult to determine what glasses prescription is needed. Eye doctors have figured out how to outsmart those muscles by paralyzing them temporarily with eyedrops. We can then prescribe exactly the glasses your child needs without underestimating or overestimating the prescription. Sometimes parents get upset at the idea of dilation because their child's vision will be blurry and the child will complain. Remember, a cycloplegic refraction is the most accurate means of prescribing glasses for children.

These dilating drops last anywhere from four to twenty-four hours and cause temporary blurring of the near vision. Reading may be difficult on the day of the examination and your child should be reassured that this is a short-term effect of the drops, but a very important part of keeping the eyes healthy.

A child's teachers should be warned that near tasks

may be difficult if the child returns to school after an examination. The child may wish to wear sunglasses, because bright lights may be bothersome.

The slit lamp is a microscope connected to a bright light. The slit lamp sits on a table and has a chin rest for your child to use while the eye doctor examines his or her eyes close up. The table has handlebars like a bike onto which your child can hold. Most children find all the buttons on the chair which go up and down fascinating, and all the instruments intriguing.

Occasionally, special tests may be needed based upon the doctor's evaluation. These tests may include color pictures of the retina and/or a fluorescein angiogram, called a dye test. Color photographs are performed at a machine similar to a slit lamp. A dye test can give valuable information about the health of the blood vessels in the retina and the health of the retina itself. Usually the dye test is ordered only in older adolescents and young adults who have had diabetes for many years.

What does a dye test, or fluorescein angiogram, consist of?

Diabetes causes damage to the retinal blood vessels and can result in closure of the vessels as well as leakage. In diabetes, the blood vessels can close off and prevent blood from flowing to vital areas of the retina. It is as though someone stepped on one of your garden hoses so patches of your lawn are yellow rather than green. In other places, the capillaries, or smallest blood vessels in the retina, may develop outpouches or microaneurysms. At these points, leakage may occur into the retina which causes swelling of the surrounding retina. The leakage is very similar to a garden hose which has many holes in it and causes water to leak all over your sidewalk.

The dye test helps determine where the leaks sprang from. The dye test can also detect areas of ischemia, or non-perfusion. These are areas where the blood vessels are so severely damaged that they are closed off. The vessels no longer supply areas of the retina with needed oxygen and nutrients; these areas of nonperfused retina correspond to the patches of yellow, parched lawn. The more severe the nonperfusion, the more likely the ophthalmologist will see signs that nonproliferative disease is severe. Severe non-proliferative disease has a high risk (more than 50 percent) of changing into proliferative disease within one year.

These areas of nonperfusion place the eye at high risk for the formation of new blood vessels which form on the surface of the retina. These new blood vessels are called neovascularization and constitute proliferative diabetic retinopathy (PDR).

New blood vessels growing to replace the diseased blood vessels sounds like a pretty good way of having the eye heal itself, right? Wrong. These new blood vessels are very detri-mental and have no useful function. Neovascularization can lead to retinal detachment (scarring in the eye pulling the retina off) and vitreous hemorrhage (bleeding inside the eye), creating a high risk of vision loss and potential blind-ness if left undiagnosed and untreated (see Chapter 3).

The dye is vegetable based and contains no iodine. It is injected into a vein using a small butterfly needle. The injection lasts ten seconds or less. The most common reaction to this test is nausea in one out of fifty people. The dye is a bright yellow and will leave the skin and urine dark yellow for about twenty-four hours.

The test requires the use of a camera and film. The film is developed in about one to two hours. Usually, the patient is allowed to return home after the test and the doctor will set up a time to discuss the results with you and decide on the next step in your child's care.

If my child has no visual symptoms, is an eye examination necessary?

Once again, children less than thirteen years of age are unlikely to have visual symptoms because of diabetes.

Diabetic retinopathy can cause damage to the retina without causing symptoms in its early stages. There are two types of vision: central and peripheral vision. Central vision is your child's reading vision—the ability to read words and see faces. Peripheral vision is your side vision—the ability to see a car passing from the side while looking straight ahead.

There are several reasons why diabetic retinopathy may go unnoticed. Diabetic retinopathy may cause the growth of new blood vessels and affect side vision before impacting central vision, or may not cause a change of vision at all.

Typically, most people use two eyes. If one eye is damaged or sees less well, this may go unnoticed unless the better-seeing eye is covered. It is rare that we close one eye to check the status of each eye separately. Hunters, however, may notice their vision is decreased when they sight a target with the dominant eye and close the nondominant eye.

What if my child complains of blurry vision? What should I do?

Blurry vision is the most common symptom reported to an eye doctor whether or not one has diabetes. There are many reasons for blurry vision in diabetics. The most common reason is elevated sugars. The excess sugar temporarily deposits itself in the natural lens within the eye and causes the lens to change shape. This transient effect is like wearing your neighbor's glasses. You don't see as well and the world appears blurry. It can take several weeks for your vision to return to normal. Glasses can help temporarily; however, when the sugars return to normal the glasses will be useless.

We recommend that you consult your pediatrician, family practitioner, or internist to help correct the cause of the elevated sugars in the first place. If the sugars are normal and the vision is blurry, an eye examination may be in order. If your child has never had an eye examination, you should consult your pediatrician, who may want to refer you to an ophthalmologist to rule out the possibility of diabetic retinopathy.

Besides retinopathy, are there other eye problems to which children and adolescents with diabetes are prone?

In general, infection among diabetics is increased. No child can avoid the common cold or occasional earache. Children with and without diabetes will get sick. Occasionally, children will develop pinkeye, or conjunctivitis, which is usually viral. You should contact your pediatrician, who may elect to refer you to an ophthalmologist for examination. Viral infections can be quite contagious. Family members should be encouraged to wash their hands frequently, not rub their eyes, and not share washcloths.

Viral eye infections are usually not treated with medicine unless there is a superimposed herpetic infection. This type of herpes is usually caused by the common cold sore and is not a form of genital herpes. In this case, the eye is often very red and can be painful; there may be vesicles or blisters on the eyelid margin. Your child usually has associated tearing and light sensitivity, and may complain of pain. He or she usually won't feel like running around and playing. This requires a specific antiviral medication for herpes.

Preseptal cellulitis is an infection of the skin around the eye and can cause swelling of the lids with a bright red color in the surrounding skin. This often needs treatment with an oral antibiotic. It can originate from a bug bite, scratch, or sinus infection. Preseptal cellulitis occurs in front of the orbital septum, or the superficial part of the lid, just beneath the skin, while orbital cellulitis occurs very deep around the eyeball itself. It can cause the skin around the eye to be very red and swollen; the eyelid often droops because of the swelling. There can be associated puslike drainage. It can be difficult to distinguish preseptal from orbital cellulitis; therefore, this diagnosis is best made by a qualified ophthalmologist.

Orbital cellulitis needs emergency evaluation, especially when it causes a change in vision, double vision, or pain with eye movement. This type of cellulitis may require hospital admission for intravenous antibiotics or surgery. Orbital cellulitis threatens vision and life.

My teenager refuses to wear glasses and now wants contact lenses. Should diabetics be allowed to wear contact lenses?

Contact lens wear in diabetics is controversial. The reason this is so is that with time, some diabetics develop a cornea which is not sensitive to pain. Pain is the unique way individuals know that a contact lens is not fitting right or is being worn for too long a period of time. Without the sensation of pain, a diabetic might develop corneal ulcers, which might ultimately threaten vision.

Some diabetics successfully wear contact lenses without difficulty. Diabetics are more prone to dry eye and infection; however, careful cleaning, disinfection, and enzyming can allow safe wear of contact lenses. Washing hands before inserting lenses combined with routine examination of the eyes to look for signs of overwear and poor fit can facilitate safe wear of lenses. This daily routine combined with close follow-up with an eye care specialist is fundamental if diabetics are going to wear contacts.

The most common causes of vision-threatening infections are improper cleaning and disinfection of lenses, sleeping in contact lenses, use of tap water with contacts, spitting on contacts, and continuing to wear contact lenses despite discomfort or development of redness. Any discomfort during contact lens wear indicates the need for prompt removal and evaluation to determine the reason for discomfort.

Can my child participate in sports, and are there any precautions for the eyes of which I should be aware?

Diabetic children can participate in all kinds of active sports. Since exercise burns up a lot of sugar, your child should have an extra snack before planned strenuous activity to avoid low blood sugar. As a rule of thumb, exercise should not be scheduled before any regular meal. Exercise should be avoided if blood sugar is ≤ 100 mg/dl or ≥ 250 mg/dl.

Coaches should be aware that your child has diabetes. They should understand the symptoms of hypoglycemia.

All children who have poor vision in one eye should use protective eyewear during any outside activity. This protective eyewear should cover both eyes and be composed of a special polycarbonate lens which resists shattering on impact; it should be prescribed by your ophthalmologist.

Is diabetic retinopathy the cause of my child's difficulty reading?

Diabetes can cause elevated sugars and blurry vision; however, if your child's sugars are now relatively normal, the likelihood that your child's difficulty reading is due to diabetic retinopathy is very low.

Diabetes rarely affects the retina at such an early age. It takes years to develop the complications of diabetic retinopathy. Many factors play a role in your child learning to read; these factors are as diverse as intelligence, hearing and speech, motivation, and visualization. Observe whether your child sits very close to the television or moves closer to the computer screen than other children. Does your child squint to see more clearly? Does one eye appear turned in or out? These may indicate a vision problem. Children may not complain like adults that their vision is blurry. Children are very adaptable and will continue playing and going to school without objection even if their vision is quite poor. They may not enjoy school, but it is rare for them to complain of poor vision.

Typically, poor vision is first picked up in the school screening examination or by a relative who asks, "why does Johnny's left eye turn in?" The most common vision problems are strabismus (cross-eye) and amblyopia (lazy eye). These are generally not related to diabetes. A child's eye becomes mature by the age of nine. Up until then, any deprivation in the eye seeing clearly becomes translated into poor vision. The eye must see crystal clear to mature properly.

The earlier a lazy eye is diagnosed, the better the prognosis for good vision. Often, the better-seeing eye must be patched to force the weaker or lazy eye to become stronger and see better. Patching can only help while the eye is in the maturation phase. After age nine, only a rare case will result in improved vision with patching or conventional treatment.

If the vision is tested and proves normal, this does not mean that your child should be able to read. Learning to read is very complex and vision is just one aspect. Many children have attention deficit disorder or dyslexia. Some parents equate these disorders with being mentally challenged; this is not the case.

The diagnosis of these conditions may need the cooperation of the teacher, the pediatrician, and other specialists. Some of the brightest children have problems with attention or dyslexia and have difficulty learning. Parents of dyslexic children themselves often had difficulty with school but were never properly diagnosed. Your child may need additional testing that may be unrelated to diabetes.

Where can I find additional support for my child and family in my local community?

The Juvenile Diabetes Foundation (JDF) was founded by parents like yourself in 1970. The Foundation has many local chapters in each state and can supply you with the latest information about the disease and ongoing research, and provide a format for you to meet other parents of children with Type I diabetes. Children can read about other children with the disease who are leading full and productive lives; they can also correspond with other kids with diabetes by regular mail or e-mail (see Appendix C).

The JDF recognizes that insulin can control diabetes but is not a cure. It actively supports diabetes research and provides significant funding for it. Its members also are politically active, campaigning for diabetes reform in health care and research. Diabetes camps exist in every state. These camps allow your child to meet other children who also have diabetes. They also teach management of diabetes and promote improved self-esteem.

Is the Internet helpful?

Computers have revolutionized the way we communicate. Many diabetes organizations are accessible via the Internet. Children with diabetes can meet other children with the disease on the "Net" and learn from their peers how to cope with chronic illness. They can learn that other children have similar interests and lead full lives. They can discover camps where children with diabetes and their friends can learn more about the disease and how to take an active role managing their own illness. Parents can learn vital information about the latest research, find the cheapest sources for purchasing syringes and glucometers, and get ready references to physicians in their area with a special interest in diabetes. The Juvenile Diabetes Foundation publishes a magazine called *Countdown* which features a special section for kids and teenagers. There is also a

special Web site for kids with diabetes. Parents should provide supervision of their children while on the Internet.

*Can children with diabetes suffer any psychological
problems?*

Diabetes can be life threatening and does complicate the
already complex process of growing up. Inevitably, diabetes will affect your child's psychosocial development.
Very young children may have difficulty in understanding
painful procedures like needle pokes and insulin injections. They may not understand why you can't make the
diabetes go away. It can be difficult to encourage good
habits and build self-esteem. It can be hard to encourage
independence and not be too overprotective.

The teen years are a particularly difficult time. This
may be one of the most difficult emotional periods for a
diabetic. Hormonal changes can aggravate diabetes, making good glucose control difficult to achieve. A child who
previously tested their sugars religiously may refuse to do
so. Food binges may become standard. Even when
teenagers use their insulin, their sugar may jump errati-
cally up and down.

They may feel the push to become independent in their
diabetes routines; however, they may be overcome with
anxiety about managing their care appropriately. The
teenage years are also a time of accepting one's own body
image. Insulin use can increase weight gain. This may conflict with images your teenager sees on TV of beautiful,
thin people with perfect jobs and lives. This conflict in
actual versus idealized body image can create a predisposition to eating disorders.

ERIC
"How a child deals with diabetes"

Eric is a five-year-old who came to us for an eye examination because his mother was also a patient of ours. Eric had started kindergarten and was really enjoying school. His mom had been very nervous about having him in school away from her watchful eye. She had met with the kindergarten teacher to show her how to use a glucometer and check Eric's sugar, although Eric was able to do this himself. They had discussed how to incorporate Eric's diabetes into the day-to-day activities of the classroom so that Eric would not feel out of place.

Eric, with the help of the teacher, did a "show and tell" about diabetes. They showed children the glucometer and used Eric's disease to help teach about the importance of healthy diets and exercise. Eric explained that sometimes his sugar goes low and he feels bad until he has a snack. Eric reported that the other kids thought the extra snacks were "pretty lucky"; however, they didn't like the part about having to poke himself all the time. Eric's mom was able to help Eric incorporate his diabetes into his classroom teaching and encouraged Eric to teach his peers about the disease. Eric's mom has certainly taken a lot of initiative to learn about the disease so she can comfortably teach her son. Sometimes a parent can feel overwhelmed with the disease and transmit this feeling to the child.

Try to give your teen as much control as possible over his or her diabetes. Discuss his or her choices and allow him or her to make as many decisions as possible. Don't be afraid to seek out additional resources, such as a diabetes educator, to help your child take as much control as possible of diabetes.

Can depression occur in diabetic children, and does this affect the eyes?

Yes. Ultimately, depression will affect the eyes.

In an ongoing ten-year study of a group of ninety-two young people who ranged in age from eight to thirteen when diagnosed with diabetes mellitus, twenty-four were diagnosed with at least one episode of clinical depression. This number is similar to the rates found in adults and is far higher than routinely found in nondiabetic children. The first year after initial diagnosis was associated with the highest incidence of depression and anxiety. Families with a history of depression should be especially alert to signs of depression.

Depression should be differentiated from momentary feelings of sadness or feeling blue. Depressed adults and children often convey feelings of pessimism, despair, guilt, and shame. They may have difficulty sleeping or sleep constantly, lose weight, have trouble concentrating, have trouble making decisions, or experience poor recent memory. They may stop enjoying activities that previously made them happy.

It is a misperception to assume that people with chronic disease should be depressed. While chronic disease has many challenges, depression is not an integral part of the disease process. Families must be aware of the higher rate of depression among diabetics and not assume children are immune. Recognizing signs of depression can help your child get the proper medical care needed to treat it. Depression is a disease just like diabetes; both can be life threatening. It is important for parents to get depressed children help because those children are vulnerable to repeated episodes of depression.

People with untreated depression are more likely to have elevated blood glucose, which inevitably leads to more complications, including diabetic retinopathy.

11

Coping with Low Vision in Diabetic Retinopathy

Diabetic retinopathy is the leading cause of new cases of blindness in the United States in patients aged twenty to sixty-four years. Through research, impressive progress is being made in the prevention and treatment of visual loss secondary to diabetes. While education and research continue to provide encouraging news, 8,000 people with diabetes will lose their sight this year and each subsequent year until a cure for diabetes is found and better emphasis on diabetic education occurs.

It can be difficult for people who are blind and diabetic to find caregivers that understand the difficulties of both blindness and diabetes. Diabetic patients often have their proliferative diabetic retinopathy successfully treated with laser treatment and/or vitrectomy. Those for whom this therapy is unsuccessful not only are disappointed with the result, but may hear, "There is nothing more that I can do." Tragically, when no referral for rehabilitative services such as low vision is forthcoming, the patient might interpret this to mean that, "Nothing more can be done." The emotional impact of this statement can be devastating.

In fact, approximately 12 percent of people referred for low-vision evaluation have diabetic retinopathy. In one study, 29 percent showed an improvement in distance prescription with an accurate refraction and 68 percent were helped with inexpensive low-vision magnifying aids.

What is legal blindness, and where did this term originate?

The definition of blindness has been debated for centuries and has undergone multiple changes based on functional impairment, economics, and total blindness. Total blindness is the inability to perceive any light. Approximately 10 percent of all those classified as legally blind are also totally blind.

The term legal blindness started out as "economic blindness" during the Great Depression, when federal projects gave millions of people employment on public works projects. Left out of this massive back-to-work project were the blind. They traditionally had been cared for by private charities, churches, their families, or by supporting themselves on the streets. During the Depression, the blind were left to fend for themselves.

The American Medical Association came up with the definition of economic blindness, or visual impairment that prevented men and women from seeing well enough to work. The Social Security Board changed the term to "legal blindness" and set numerical visual measurements as a basis for eligibility for financial and other benefits.

The term legal blindness is considered outdated by

many in the United States and in some countries. It defines legal blindness as corrected visual acuity of 20/200 or less and a field of 20 degrees or less; it does not consider a person's functional ability—how well he or she is able to perform daily activities with or without visual aids.

Do all legally blind people have the same bad vision?

No. Legal blindness is a spectrum of decreased vision defined currently by a minimum standard.

The term legal blindness is disputed by many low-vision specialists because it overestimates the number of legally blind individuals. The majority of legally blind people are actually partially sighted. They are able, with the help of appropriate visual aids, to read ordinary printed material, live independently, write with pen and pencil, and walk without a cane, guide dog, or sighted companion. Most partially sighted people will never become functionally blind.

What is low vision, and how did the field develop?

Low vision means that a person wearing regular glasses or contact lenses can't read the newspaper, see a friend's face, read street signs, or see the labels in a grocery store. In adults, the major causes of low vision are diabetic retinopathy, age-related macular degeneration, and glaucoma. In children, the major causes are amblyopia (lazy eye), strabismus (cross-eye), cataracts, injuries, and, less commonly, retinal conditions such as retinopathy of prematurity (a disease of premature babies).

In the late 1950s, many doctors, surgeons, and optical

specialists shifted their emphasis from blindness to sight-edness by advocating research and development of new ways to measure vision and new devices to rehabilitate the partially sighted, maximizing the use of whatever existing vision a patient had.

When should I see a low-vision specialist, and will my eye doctor refer me when I am ready?

There is no magic level of vision that determines when to send you to a low-vision specialist. Just as diabetes affects each person differently, so each person is unique in his or her visual needs. Loss of vision is defined as poor vision that can't be corrected with a lens. You might be 20/200 without glasses but 20/20 with glasses. This is not what we mean by low vision or vision loss. Visual distortion means that letters might be wavy or lines distorted. Vision is not merely how well you read the eye chart. Vision is very complex. The eye chart is a gross estimate of your vision and does not measure your ability to contrast and see colors. It also doesn't measure your reading speed.

I have had patients with 20/20 vision who are distressed by some letters being black and others being gray, or noting letters missing in words. I have had other patients with 20/200 vision who feel life is great and their vision is fine—"I get about fine and I see the TV fine." Each person's visual requirements vary. This is why it is so important to convey to your eye doctor in general how you are doing with your vision. Many diabetics report having "good vision days" and "bad vision days." Others report that positioning their glasses differently allows them to see better . . . taking them off to read, sliding them down the nose, or tilting them forward. These are all common maneuvers that suggest your vision might be improved with a new prescription.

If you have vision loss that can't be corrected and you are having difficulty writing checks, reading books, or with any daily household tasks such as grocery shopping, reading recipe books, or reading the fine print in papers, it is probably time for a low-vision referral. Being referred to a low-vision doctor has yet to become a reflex among all eye care practitioners. I wish each one would take the time to ask about how you are adapting to your vision loss. Don't be afraid to ask your doctor about low-vision devices. He or she may refer you to a low-vision specialist. Remember, low vision is a rapidly developing field and is more complex than just recommending a magnifier.

One of my patients, a forty-four-year-old woman, developed 20/200 vision from diabetic macular edema. Her diabetes and blood pressure had been poorly controlled and were just now becoming regulated. She was frustrated with her current vision and had tried over-the-counter magnifiers. She had a very supportive family and a brother who was a physician. We had instituted every measure including laser to treat her macular edema; however, her medical condition had been so unstable over the years that eventually, vision loss slowly ensued. She grew increasingly intolerant of her diabetes and frustrated with her visual difficulties.

We encouraged her to see a low-vision specialist; we thought she would benefit because she was motivated to be able to perform certain visual tasks. Different aids were tried, and a few were found to be helpful. She appreciated a higher-plus bifocal in addition to a very high-powered magnifier (24x). She liked the yellow tint used to diminish glare and improve contrast. She also found the talking glucometer helpful as well as the talking watch. She learned about community services available to the visually impaired, such as talking books, phone services, and less expensive city bus fares. She thanked us for referring her to the low-vision specialist because she became aware of other available resources in case her vision became worse.

What should a person expect from a visit to a low-vision specialist?

Before you visit a low-vision specialist, you must understand that this visit is very different from visiting the family doctor. Low-vision specialists are eager to help you achieve your visual goals. To do this, you must be specific about the visual activities that are important to you. Difficulty communicating which visual tasks are significant may prevent the low-vision specialist from helping you accomplish these activities.

A low-vision aid is any device which helps a partially sighted individual see more clearly and function more efficiently. A common misconception about low-vision aids is that they cure the damaging eye disease of diabetes. Because the eye behaves like a camera, and the damage from diabetes occurs in the retina or film part of a camera, changing the lens on the front of the camera does not fix the damaged retina. Low-vision aids merely enhance your current usable vision.

Low-vision devices are tailored to specific tasks. A device that works well for quick reading of labels in the grocery store may not be well suited for long-term reading of books or magazines. A magnifier on a stand may help for writing checks, but may not be strong enough for books.

Thus, it is crucial for individuals to think carefully about their goals for vision rehabilitation.

Compile a list of goals for vision rehabilitation by thinking about your daily routine.

❖ Do you have trouble preparing meals?

❖ Are you able to work and drive to work?

❖ If you work, are you able to complete your job responsibilities in an efficient manner?

❖ If you drive, are you able to see street signs?

❖ Are you able to read mail, write letters, balance your checkbook?

❖ Are there books or magazines or correspondence that you have trouble reading?

❖ Can you see TV well enough to follow the action?

❖ When you shop, can you read labels, prices, and aisle signs?

❖ Does your job require you to read a computer, fax, or copier display?

❖ Are you able to read a menu?

❖ Can you read train, bus, and airline flight schedules?

❖ Are you able to enjoy your work activities and hobbies?

❖ Are you comfortable crossing a busy street?

Once you have identified the problem areas, make a list of specific visual tasks you find difficult and bring in examples of print that is difficult for you to read. These might include a Bible, handwritten letters, bills and bank statements, recipes, stock exchange listings, and the newspaper. Now you and the low-vision specialist can begin exploring possible solutions. You might end up with several devices, each of which is best suited for a different specific activity.

To best understand how the low-vision specialist can help you, you will be asked about the onset of your vision loss, your family history of vision loss, and particularly about your medications. Some eyedrops can affect your pupil size and accommodative ability, or ability to read close up. Unless the doctor knows about your medications, he may be misled by unequal pupil sizes, color vision disorders, double vision, or increased sensitivity to light.

The first part of the assessment is a full exam which includes a refraction (checking the glasses prescription). Near, intermediate, and distance vision are checked. It is very important that you bring all glasses and magnifiers you are using with you to the examination. Do not expect the doctor to prescribe a new pair of glasses right away. Diabetes can cause fluctuations in vision because of swelling in the retina or changes in the sugar level affecting the natural lens in the eye. Your doctor may wait to ensure that your prescription is stable for at least two visits before prescribing a pair of glasses. Your doctor is trying to save you the added expense of prescribing the wrong pair of glasses for you.

A dilated examination might be included if the doctor or one of his associates has not evaluated the reason for decreased vision. A dilated examination is always indicated if your visual acuity has changed significantly from a previous visit or assessment. Be prepared to be dilated at the initial visit. The low-vision specialist needs to know whether the damage to your retina is old or progressive and whether it is the entire reason for your visual impairment. After the doctor completes the clinical examination, the doctor and patient can begin to explore possible solutions tailored to individual visual tasks. Various low-vision aids will be tested.

Low-vision devices are categorized into near devices, distance devices, electronic devices, and nonoptical devices. Corning protective filters (CPF) and sunlenses, usually in the yellow wavelength, have been found to be helpful in improving contrast and eliminating glare and photophobia. Direct illumination, especially for near tasks, is generally beneficial. A flashlight is helpful if a patient is experiencing poor night vision. Near devices include handheld magnifiers, high-powered reading glasses, and telescopes focused for near. Unlike the long telescopes used to view the stars in the sky, near telescopes are miniaturized ones a few inches long and no wider than a half dollar. Some of these can be mounted in a pair of glasses. The main function of most low-vision telescopes is distance magnification, but some can be focused near.

Electronic devices include closed circuit television (CCTV) and the Magni-Cam™. The CCTV is a zoom lens which can be focused on reading material. The material is then displayed on a screen. By adjusting various controls on the closed circuit television, the letters can be made larger and smaller and the color of the letters and background can be varied.

Non-optical devices include writing aids such as bold-lined paper and guides to help with writing checks and addressing envelopes, stands, colored acetate filters (clear sheets of colored plastic that may enhance contrast and reduce glare), large-print publications, and special dials for televisions and stoves (see Figure 11.1). Other aids include the glucose monitor with talking reader and

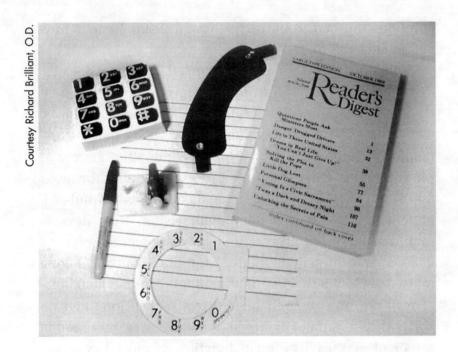

Courtesy Richard Brilliant, O.D.

Figure 11.1 **Non-optical devices: large print** Reader's Digest, **numbered phone dials (rotary and push button), needle threader, felt-tip pen (for darker, bolder print), and visor that attaches to a patient's spectacle frames**

insulin syringe aids to assist with measuring the right amount of insulin.

An eye specialist may not show you a particular low-vision aid because he or she knows in advance that it probably won't work for you. For example, some people have an uncontrollable tremor or crippling arthritis that prevents them from comfortably using small, handheld devices. The low-vision specialist may bypass a small handheld magnifier in favor of a stand magnifier which does not require that one steadies the material oneself (see Figure 11.2).

Make sure you understand how each device works before you make any decisions about which one is best for you. Have a realistic idea of which tasks you can accomplish with the device. Some low-vision centers will even allow you to borrow a device for home use for a few days or weeks before making a decision. After you express your

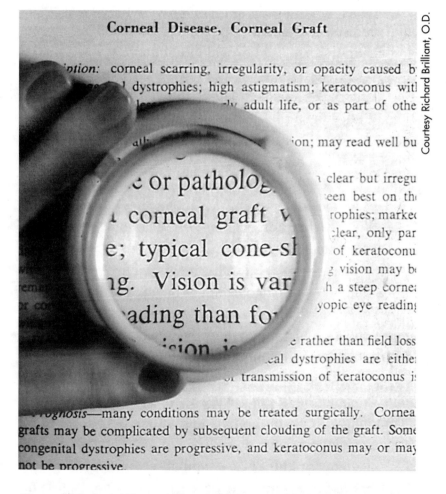

Figure 11.2 A stand magnifier provides a stable base and may be easier to use for some patients than a handheld magnifier.

preferences, the doctor will order and dispense them to you. He will wish to schedule a follow-up appointment to see how well the device is working for you.

Do not expect a low-vision specialist to prescribe contact lenses or progressive lenses (bifocals without a line) to you. Contact lenses for diabetics are controversial. Diabetes can affect nerves, and the cornea, or covering of the eye is no exception. Its nerves can become desensitized and predispose the diabetic to breakdown of the cornea and vision-threatening corneal infection.

Progressive lenses work by having graduated power in the center of the lens as you look down in the reading position. While these glasses are cosmetically preferable to many, the peripheral distortion, sometimes called swimming, can be an added nuisance for someone with already impaired vision.

The low-vision evaluation can be time consuming. It takes a while to explore all these options; some people prefer to make several visits. Being tired can prevent you from determining the best option for rehabilitating your vision.

Not all your visual goals might be achieved with a low-vision specialist. For example, if traveling on foot in a safe manner is a problem, you may need the services of an orientation and mobility instructor. Another type of specialist, a rehabilitation teacher, may be needed if you have difficulty using the stove, using medications like insulin, matching clothing, and other daily tasks. If your problem is maintaining your job, the specialist may refer you to the state agency for the visually impaired for career placement and job assistance. If peer support is an issue, you may be referred to a support group in your area.

Why should I attend a low-vision support group?

Many patients have found low-vision support groups invaluable. Initially, many of my patients laugh at the idea of going to a low-vision support group. They associate it with being emotionally needy or depressed. These groups are free; there is nothing to lose by attending. A low-vision support group can supply you with the latest invaluable information about your disease, managing low vision, accomplishing tasks which are visually difficult, and the pros and cons of various low-vision devices from firsthand users. They can even offer advice ranging from tax tips to transportation discounts for the visually impaired. Attending a support group means you want to learn more about your disease and maximize your usable vision. It helps to have some encouragement.

Vision loss is a major life crisis, and like any crisis, adaptation is needed. The more supportive friends and family you have, the better. Support can also be found outside in people with a similar visual impairment. Outsiders who have not heard the story of your vision loss can sometimes be more sympathetic to your visual rehabilitation. People who have undergone the same day-to-day problems can offer guidance and useful information ranging from referrals to knowledgeable physicians to low-vision devices to good nutritional support. As with any support group, it is best to attend at least two sessions before deciding whether you should join the group.

Support groups and information can also be found in your own home via the Internet. Feel free to "surf the Net" by searching such key phrases as diabetic retinopathy, diabetes, and low vision. You can enter "chat rooms" to discuss diabetes anonymously (see Appendix C).

Should I worry about my diabetic child needing low-vision help?

No. Diabetes is a rare cause of visual impairment or vision loss in children. Adolescents are the youngest children to develop diabetic retinopathy of any type. While low-vision services exist for infants, toddlers, and children of any age, the cause will not be diabetes.

What is the Magni-Cam™, and is it useful to people like myself with central vision loss from diabetic retinopathy?

The Magni Cam™ is a small, portable magnification system which has been available for several years. People who benefit from magnification up to 25x are most likely to be helped by this device. People with diabetic retinopathy and age-related macular degeneration who have lost central vision are most likely to be aided. Several options to increase portability are available.

The Magni-Cam™ itself is composed of a handheld camera unit with a built-in fluorescent light source, so you can scan over text (see Figure 11.3). The camera unit can be connected to three different sources for viewing the enlarged text. The camera can be connected to your television set to provide a monochrome video image. The magnification provided is approximately double the diagonal size of the television screen. For example, a 25-inch TV screen would provide up to 50x magnification. Curved surfaces like cans and pill bottles can be imaged without blur, unlike closed circuit television cameras (CCTVs). Like a CCTV, the camera has a knob to allow contrast adjustment, and reverse contrast can change print to white on a black background.

A second option is to connect the camera to a 6-inch display top which is similar to a laptop computer screen. This offers portability and allows you to take the camera out shopping; it provides up to 25x magnification. The last option is a head-mounted display which weighs about 7 ounces and provides up to 25x magnification. Prescription glasses can be worn under the device. In the market, you can place the eyepieces above your eyes and reposition them over your eyes when you need to read a price or label. Power is provided by a rechargeable battery pack or by plugging directly into an electrical outlet.

Advantages of the Magni-Cam™ are portability and depth of focus. You can read and write with the Magni-Cam™, but you can also take it with you while you shop or

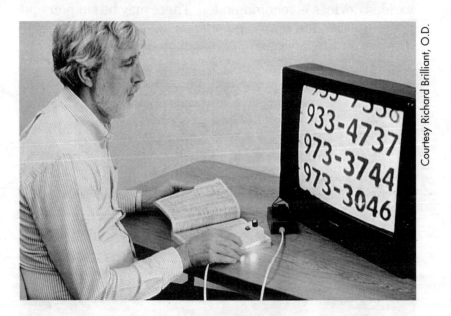

Courtesy Richard Brilliant, O.D.

Figure 11.3 The Magni-Cam™ (manufactured by Innoventions, Inc., Littleton, Colorado) is one type of CCTV in which the camera is handheld and can be attached to a television set.

travel. The Magni-Cam™ is not designed to see distant objects. The disadvantages of the Magni-Cam™ include the necessity to have a steady hand and physically move the camera across a line. In some diabetics, peripheral neuropathy may make this difficult. A CCTV, however, does not require such a steady hand. The LVES, or low-vision enhancement system (see Figure 11.4), can be used to zoom in and magnify objects at any distance in black and white; however, it weighs more than a Magni-Cam™. The cost of a Magni-Cam™ is around $700. The battery pack and portable attachments are an additional cost. The LVES is considerably more expensive.

Before considering purchasing any low-vision device, a thorough evaluation by a low-vision specialist and trial of various devices is recommended. There may be simpler and more cost-effective aids that meet your individual needs.

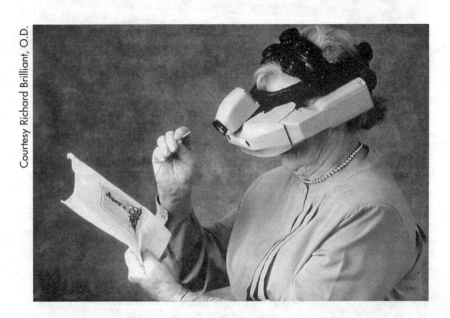

Courtesy Richard Brilliant, O.D.

Figure 11.4 **The low-vision enhancement system (LVES)**

Some low-vision centers will let you borrow a device prior to making an expensive purchase. Take advantage of an offer to try a device in your own home for a few weeks.

How am I supposed to read my glucometer if I can't see?

Several products are available to assist in using insulin. Microscopes or high-power reading glasses allow magnification but leave your hands free to draw up the insulin. These can be prescribed by a low-vision specialist. Syringes with large numbers are especially useful when the syringe is placed in front of a contrasting background (see Figure 11.5). Syringes with stops which prevent you from drawing up an excessive amount are also available. The only problem with these syringes is determining whether the insulin contains air bubbles. There are also adapters which connect to the glucometer and read the glucose

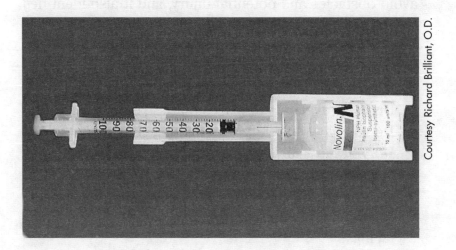

Courtesy Richard Brilliant, O.D.

Figure 11.5 Non-optical gauges are helpful for patients who cannot see markings on their insulin syringe obtain the correct dosage.

level out loud, and blood pressure cuffs which read aloud the numbers for the visually impaired. Magnifiers are also available that attach to the glucometer; however, the amount of magnification is usually low (around 2x).

Why do people walk with a cane, and when should you get a white cane?

There are special classes offered by orientation and mobility instructors to enhance independent travel. After you have been evaluated by a low-vision specialist to determine whether your vision can be improved with glasses or magnifiers, you may undergo visual rehabilitation which can include "learning to walk again," either with a white cane or possibly with a seeing guide dog.

The purpose of using a cane is twofold. It helps a blind person to move independently and more safely, and to avoid obstacles and potential injury, and it also identifies the individual as visually impaired to automobiles.

If you answer yes to any of the following questions, you may want to consider learning cane travel.

❖ Do you miss elevation changes like steps or curbs?
❖ Do you travel only to places that are familiar to you?
❖ Do you have difficulty with lighting changes?
❖ Do you have difficulty interpreting shadows or other color changes in walking surfaces?
❖ Do you spend a lot of time looking down at the ground?
❖ Do you bump into obstacles like coffee tables or door facings?

Cane training can be very extensive and may require up to 160 hours. The length of training can be adjusted to suit the needs and lifestyle of the student. Training can be conducted in various settings and situations that the student uses daily.

Does vision loss affect your other senses: smell, touch, taste, hearing?

Vision loss has not made your other senses sharper; however, you utilize and rely more heavily upon them than you did before.

Walk along a busy street and hear the end of the building line. A building reflects and blocks sound, but as you arrive at the intersection, the full effect of the city should be heard. The natural elements are no longer blocked by buildings and you can feel the wind and sun beat against you. Hear the truck as it passes by and know the direction of the traffic.

Sound quickly falls away in small rooms and softens in large open spaces. Listen quietly in a room to the sounds—the refrigerator motor intermittently kicks in, the computer hums and keys click, the air conditioner hums, the clock ticks on the mantelpiece, the birds chirp outside the window. The examples of sound guiding are endless and environment dependent.

In the grocery store, the senses of smell and touch are invaluable. Feel the shape of the fruit as well as feel for soft spots. Estimate weight. Smell the sweetness of the fruit. In a workshop, organize nails, screws, and washers by their shapes. Place them into small containers for easy identification and put an example of each on the outside of the container with a piece of tape.

Adapting to nonvisual clues does not occur overnight.

Nonvisual clues are abundant and take some practice to read. With patience and study, the confidence that comes from having an accurate picture of what is happening around you will develop.

How do your other senses help with daily activities?

Hearing helps you recognize friends and family by their voices or footsteps. Listening to the tone of their voices will help you detect anger, joy, irritation, and disappointment. An enthusiastic greeting comes with a smile. Listen to the sound of traffic. It lets you know whether it is safe to cross the street.

Utilize talking devices such as watches, calculators, and scales. Use a liquid level detector so that you stop pouring when you hear the beep. Record recipes on tape in alphabetical order so that you have a way of listening while you prepare meals.

When cooking, pay attention to the sounds of food. Listen to the loud bubbling noise that becomes louder and faster as liquid boils. When frying food, listen to the pop that lets you know food is browning. When the sounds die down, the food is usually ready to be turned.

Touching helps you recognize the texture of clothes and distinguish cotton, linen, silk, and wool. Feeling distinguishing characteristics such as buttons, zippers, collars, and pockets can help you identify which item of clothing you have selected. Trace the shape of items like shoes and earrings.

Use your sense of smell to locate a restaurant and use that as an orientation point. Large department stores often have colognes and perfumes located at an entrance; use this as an orientation point.

What are some home improvement tips that can help me maximize my vision?

Porcelain, tile, and linoleum are shiny and can increase glare in a bright room. Consider curtains for windows and a dimmer switch for lighting. Don't wax linoleum floors; you will only increase glare. Unpatterned flooring in the bathroom is best, since it is less distracting and can help make dropped items easier to find. Corners and edges of rugs should be tacked or taped down to prevent tripping. Paint the threshold of doorways bright colors to prevent tripping.

In the bathroom, use cups, soap dishes, and a toothbrush of a contrasting color to the countertop. Select a toothbrush with a dark handle which contrasts with the white bristles to help you place the toothpaste. Install a wall-mounted soap dispenser to maintain a constant location. Install a wall-mounted mirror with an extension mirror and magnifying mirror to assist with shaving or make-up application. Organize, organize, organize. Place extra shelves, organizers, and dividers in drawers, cabinets, and cupboards to help sort items.

In medicine cabinets, alphabetize and return containers to their places when done. Use large-lettered labels on look-alike bottles. Place one or two rubber bands around important medications.

To avoid hitting your head on cabinets, when you open one remove the item and close it promptly. Teach other family members to do the same. Paint your cabinet a bright or contrasting color. Change to sliding doors.

In the bathtub, to avoid overfilling, use a colorful float toy to mark the water level. To assure that the water temperature is just right, mark the control knob with a dot of nail polish at the desired adjustment. Avoid scalding by running cold water, then adding hot. If you have a sliding-glass door on your bath or shower, decorate it with brightly colored stickers for safety. Nonslip guards for the bottom of your tub are an excellent idea. Contrasting bath towels also help. Consider soap on a rope or brightly colored soap bars. Similarly, reusable colored plastic bottles are ideal for shampoo, conditioner, and other bath products. A permanent waterproof marker can be used to show the contents of each bottle. Pump dispensers work equally well to help organize the bath. Use contrast right down to the toilet paper and toilet seat.

12

Depression, Diabetes, and Blindness

"STOP." To many diabetics, the world looks like a giant stop sign full of do's and don'ts. Making life even more difficult are the "diabetes police"—people without diabetes who enjoy pointing out these do's and don'ts. "Did the doctor tell you that was OK to eat?" "Shouldn't you check your sugar now?" Those of us without diabetes sometimes try to create "perfect diabetic" patients by insisting unrealistically that they adopt the Ten Commandments: "Thou shalt . . ."

1. Take insulin and pills at the right time.
2. Exercise daily.
3. Avoid fatty foods.
4. Avoid smoking or drinking alcohol.
5. Avoid sweets or sugars (if you eat them then you're a cheater).
6. Stick to the meal plan no matter how bland.

7. Check blood sugar levels several times each day and adjust blood sugar so that it never runs high or low.
8. Stay on the alert at all times for signs of low sugar.
9. Keep blood pressure perfect.
10. Keep the regimen day in and day out forever.

We all know that the perfect diabetic cannot exist. This is not from lack of real effort on many patients' parts, but medical science has yet to devise a way to reduplicate the actions of the pancreas. Living with diabetes is not easy. Inevitably, there will be good days when your glucose is rock stable and there will be bad days when your sugar jumps high and low with no discernible reason for the fluctuation. There may be frustrating days when you can't stop eating, when you can't get motivated to exercise, or when you step on the bathroom scale and notice weight gain. There may be upsetting and frightening days when a minor or major complication develops. Living with chronic disease means that one will normally experience many emotions over the long term. When depression and anxiety become the constant mood, medical help may be needed. Depression, anxiety, and eating disorders are common among diabetic patients. These can lead to poor glucose control, which can ultimately affect the eyes.

Many depressive episodes have a biochemical basis just like high blood pressure. Our country still is reluctant to recognize depression as a legitimate disease. Medical science has discovered many important chemicals in our brains which, when out of balance, can cause depression. There is a biological basis for depression. Depression can be life threatening. It is extremely important to understand that your psychological health is just as important as your kidney function and your eyesight. It is perhaps more difficult to measure. You can help yourself or a family member you care about by getting medical attention for emotional imbalances.

Is depression associated with diabetes?

Depression is common with any chronic illness, especially one which you must confront every day at mealtime. Fifteen to 20 percent of diabetic patients, both Type I and Type II, in the United States suffer from serious depression—a rate approximately three times the general population. Over a lifetime, 35 to 40 percent of diabetics will have a major depressive episode at least once. A major depressive episode is one which interferes with daily functioning, interpersonal relationships, and family life.

There are many factors that predispose one to depression, such as family history, medications, and environmental factors. Many diabetics are predisposed to problems with impotence which can lead to added stress in a marriage and even trigger depression. Pervasive stress and strain may cause depression for the family member with diabetes. Parents who are depressed or anxious can pass this on to children with diabetes as a learned behavior.

When complications like diabetic retinopathy develop, new bouts of depression might be triggered, especially among people who have struggled to avoid complications throughout the duration of their diabetes. In one study, 68 percent of patients with blindness from diabetic retinopathy reported severe depression at least once.

What are the signs of depression?

A common screening test for depression is the Beck Depression Inventory. Experiencing some of these symptoms may indicate that you need further evaluation for possible depression. Any concerns about depression should be addressed with a health care professional.

❖ hopelessness
❖ sense of failure
❖ lack of pleasure
❖ weight loss
❖ trouble concentrating
❖ trouble with decision making
❖ lack of energy or enthusiasm
❖ sadness, pessimism, or despair
❖ guilt and shame
❖ crying spells
❖ self-blame
❖ fatigue
❖ sleeplessness, insomnia
❖ excessive sleeping
❖ disinterest in work
❖ inability to work
❖ loss of appetite
❖ lack of interest in people
❖ suicidal thoughts

Failure to take insulin, check blood sugars, and take medications can be responses to depression. Depression in diabetics has been consistently linked to all kinds of problems that have negative effects on glucose control—obesity, smoking, alcohol abuse, physical inactivity, and nonadherence to a daily regimen. It's hard to tell which comes first: the poor control or the depression. The link between the two—diabetes and depression—has led researchers to investigate whether a chemical in the brain might be responsible.

Suicidal thoughts often indicate severe depression: "My family would be better off if I were not alive" or, "No matter what I do my diabetes gets worse; I want to die and get this over with." Suicidal thoughts indicate severe depression and need emergency attention. There are various degrees of depression, and it can be short- or long-term. Being sad is different from being depressed. Sadness and disappointment are normal, everyday emotions. However, if sadness is associated with other symptoms, it can be linked to depression. Depression is an illness that often requires treatment but unfortunately often goes unrecognized.

Depressive episodes can last for months. If untreated, these episodes are more likely to recur once, twice, or more in a patient's lifetime. Diabetics at highest risk are those with a family history of depression. Lots of stress and strain in daily life can also put a diabetic at increased risk. New bouts of depression can be triggered by new complications.

Is "talk therapy" a substitute for medication?

Talk therapy is not a substitute for antidepressant medications if a diabetic patient is severely depressed. Besides taking your normal diabetic medications, specific medical treatment for depression is necessary and should be initiated by a care provider with expertise in this area. Various

ANDREW
"The vicious cycle of depression"

Andrew was a fifty-eight-year-old man who had recently
lost considerable vision from macular edema and macular ischemia. He was a new patient to me. Looking back
through his chart, there were several missed appointments in a row, and he had not been seen for a full year.
I asked him how he'd been coping with his diabetes and
mentioned that some of my patients occasionally had
rough times with the disease. I could tell he was not a
talkative person, so we just stuck with the basics. He told
me that his vision was worse, and he could no longer
read the paper. He was angry about having worse vision
even though he had received laser treatment.

I took the time to review his fluorescein angiograms
on a magnified light box so he could see the damage
from the diabetes and how the laser had helped. I
explained that some of the damage had not been fixable. He asked point-blank if missing his appointments
had caused him to lose more vision. Beating a man
when he's down never helps, so I simply told him that
sometimes patients miss appointments for legitimate
reasons. He then explained that his wife had died, and
he now lived by himself without any family. He lost his
job because he "just couldn't get up in the morning."
He couldn't cook, and he now ate terribly. He added
that he had no appetite. He stopped taking his medications because he had no interest in life. He jokingly
asked for the phone number of Dr. Kevorkian. He had
only kept his appointment with us today because his

optometrist had refused to give him new glasses until he saw a retinal specialist. I asked Andrew honestly whether he'd really considered taking his own life. "If I had more energy," he responded.

We asked the hospital social worker to meet with Andrew before we let him go home because he had many of the signs of severe depression. His blood sugar measured 350 mg/dl in our office (110 mg/dl is normal). His blood pressure was also very high. He had no insurance because he had lost his job, and he had stopped getting medical care. Depression was having a cyclic effect.

A psychiatrist, with the help of a social worker, met with Andrew immediately and assessed him. She prescribed the medication Zoloft for depression and made appointments to meet with him regularly. A resident interested in diabetes offered to provide Andrew with the medical care he needed and he was restarted on his insulin regimen. A dietitian met with him at the hospital to teach him about which foods to eat. Andrew learned how to cook some simple nutritional dishes. For three months, we were able to get his diabetic medications from an assistance program for the needy sponsored by the drug company that makes the medications. In this time, his personality completely changed. He found a job working in a sports store as a general manager. He eventually agreed to see a low-vision specialist for help with his near vision. Andrew is now doing extremely well and has been closely followed with the help of his psychiatrist. He also participates in the local hospital's diabetes support group.

talk therapies can be helpful to teach specific skills and coping mechanisms but they are not a substitute for medication in severe depression. However, talk therapy may be effective for mild depression.

For example, interpersonal therapy helps patients deal with family problems and relationships. Cognitive behavior therapy is another form of psychotherapy that can be beneficial.

Any health care professional, including your eye specialist, can refer you to a specialist in depression such as a psychiatrist. You should feel free to discuss depression with any of your care providers. Your insurance may require your internist to refer you to a mental health care professional just as an internist might refer you to a cardiologist if you had a complex heart problem.

What kinds of medications are used to treat depression in diabetics?

A group of antidepressant medications called selective serotonin reuptake inhibitors (SSRIs) are commonly prescribed. These medications include Zoloft, Paxil, Prozac, and Vuxol. As a group, these medications tend to promote weight loss and decrease the insulin dose, especially among obese individuals with diabetes, as well as combat depression. It can take several weeks to see significant benefit from the medications and the dosage may need to be slowly increased to achieve maximum benefit. Because they do not provide immediate gratification, these medications are not habit forming. These same medications are also used to treat eating disorders.

Are medications to treat depression safe to use for diabetics?

In one study, patients who were treated with the antidepressant nortryptiline showed significant improvement in their glucose control in just over eight weeks. The one side effect of Nortryptiline was unexpected hyperglycemic effects. Newer drugs to fight depression are proving equally effective without the elevated glucose side effect. Ask your doctor whether your antidepressant medication causes elevated glucose. If it does, your diabetes medication may need to be adjusted.

The most common antidepressants prescribed are serotonin reuptake inhibitors (such as Prozac, Zoloft, and Paxil). These medications are not habit forming, but they do need to be monitored. The dose may have to be adjusted for maximum effectiveness and minimum side effects, which can include hypoglycemia (low blood sugar) and weight loss.

Are there any risk factors for depression?

A family history of depression indicates a genetic predisposition. Environmental factors can play a role in families in which diabetes is present. Constant stress and strain creates a much higher risk of the diabetic developing depression.

What are the known medical causes of depression which contribute to depression in diabetes?

There are many medical conditions which can cause depression. Neurological conditions, infections, and rheumatological conditions have also been linked to depression.

CARL
"Surgery and depression"

Another patient, Carl, had severe proliferative diabetic retinopathy in addition to a host of medical
problems which included high blood pressure, kidney
failure necessitating dialysis three times a week, and
neuropathy requiring a walking foot cast. He had had
the maximum amount of laser treatment for his proliferative diabetic retinopathy and macular edema. The
proliferation of blood vessels continued despite our
best efforts. The next step was vitrectomy surgery to
remove the jelly (vitreous) in both eyes. Despite all this,
he was cheerful and explained that "the man upstairs
had it all under control."

After the surgery in his left eye, he was thrilled.
He saw a low-vision specialist and was able to read
again with the help of an 18x magnifier. His great joy
in life was attending church on Sunday. Now he could
read parts of the hymnal. I knew Carl as a happy and
jovial man. One day his wife called frantically saying
that Carl was having "an attack of nerves" and could
see nothing. He came to the office with a vitreous hemorrhage, or bleeding into the eye. He could only see
my hand move in front of his face. We performed an
ultrasound which showed that the retina was in its
proper place behind the blood. We reassured him that
the blood would likely disappear on its own. His blood
pressure that day was extremely high—220/115.

He was subsequently admitted to the hospital because of his severe blood pressure. During this time, the blood inside his left eye began to plug the drain in his eye, causing the eye pressure to rise dangerously high. We treated the eye pressure with multiple glaucoma drops; however, this was unsuccessful. Over a week's time, the kidney, heart, and general doctors had little success bringing his blood pressure down. Carl grew more and more disappointed and frustrated in the hospital. He also reported being exhausted by all the hospital tests and treatments around the clock. Carl's pastor visited daily for long periods of time and was able to keep Carl full of hope.

We explained to Carl that he would need to have another vitrectomy in his left eye to wash out the blood so that the eye pressure could normalize again. He refused the surgery until he could "go home, sleep in my own bed, and go to church on Sunday." While Carl seemed depressed, he had not lost hope. He believed that if he could sleep in his own bed and go to church that the surgery would be successful. His renal doctor let him go home and we performed a successful surgery the following Monday. Carl was elated at his improved vision and is now doing extremely well. We did not feel that Carl was acutely depressed. He had an excellent support network and seemed to react appropriately to all the stresses of hospitalization.

Endocrine disorders which affect the thyroid, parathyroid, and adrenal glands can cause it. Postpartum depression can occur. Many medications have been linked to depression: heart medications, blood pressure medications, antibiotics, anti-inflammatory medications, chemotherapeutic medications, sedatives, anti-Parkinson medications, and steroids. This is why it is important to be familiar with the side effects of all your medications so that side effects such as depression can be minimized.

Do children with diabetes suffer depression?

Yes. In one ongoing study of ninety-two children age eight to thirteen, twenty-four were diagnosed with at least one episode of clinical depression. This is similar to the rate in adults and far higher than in children without diabetes. The first year after initial diagnosis was associated with the highest incidence of depression or anxiety disorders. It is important for parents to get help for depressed children because they are vulnerable to repeated episodes during adulthood. (See Chapter 10 on childhood diabetes.)

Are eating disorders common in diabetes and can they affect the eye?

Diabetic women have higher levels of eating disorder attitudes and behavior than the general population. Eating disorders such as anorexia nervosa and bulimia nervosa are rare in diabetics. Uncontrollable binge eating, intense preoccupation with weight, and intentional insulin omission are heartbreakingly familiar among diabetic women who live in our society that idolizes the thin model. The medical consequences of eating disorders in diabetes can be devastating. Diabetic retinopathy is markedly increased in diabetic patients with eating disorders.

Standard diabetes care focuses on diet and exercise. This focus on weight, eating, and exercise may place women with Type I diabetes at risk for developing a preoccupation with body shape and inappropriate dieting habits. Adolescence is a time of heightened awareness of weight, shape, and body image. Because many Type I diabetics are diagnosed in preadolescence and adolescence, young women with diabetes are more likely to struggle with disordered eating than their peers.

The potential to misuse insulin as a means of controlling weight gain is ever present. One patient may decrease her insulin dose to promote the spilling of calories in the urine or omit a dose completely. Another may fail to increase her insulin to compensate for an episode of binge eating in order to avoid weight gain. These actions promote hyperglycemia and poor glucose control, and contribute to long-term complications.

Treatment focuses on a mixture of psychotherapy to help change eating habits and improve glucose control and antidepressant medication such as selective serotonin inhibitors (SSRIs). SSRIs have been shown to result in modest weight loss and decreases in insulin requirement.

The DCCT recommended intensive therapy and tight control to reduce the risk of complications like retinopathy in Type I diabetics. However, weight gain is a consequence of such intensive insulin therapy. Insulin promotes sugar uptake into your body tissues where it can be used for energy. Any woman with intense concerns about weight or body shape may have trouble with intensive insulin therapy. Acknowledging concerns about body image and seeking counseling may also be helpful. Alternatively, insulin pump therapy, which traditionally requires less insulin, may help offset weight gain associated with intensive therapy.

Can depression and eating disorders lead to eye complications?

Depression has been consistently linked to all kinds of negative outcomes: smoking, obesity, alcohol abuse, and physical inactivity. Depression can affect a patient's ability to care for himself or herself. This includes blood glucose monitoring, administering insulin, taking other medications, and keeping appointments. Lack of attention to these matters can lead to poor glucose control, which is the major mechanism of diabetic complications. Eating disorders can also contribute to poor glucose control.

Is blindness associated with depression?

In one survey, 68 percent of all diabetics with total blindness reported at least one bout of major depression. Any visual impairment involves loss and can lead to anger, denial, and depression. Professional help from physicians, counselors, and low-vision support groups, along with visual rehabilitation may successfully combat depression. However, because depression often has a biological basis, medication may be necessary to help deal with it, in conjunction with a supportive environment.

NANCY
"Medication-induced depression"

Nancy is a thirty-eight-year-old insulin dependent diabetic who I followed because of her proliferative diabetic retinopathy. She is generally a friendly, gregarious, and outgoing person who believes in taking her diabetes "one day at a time." Her blood pressure was elevated in our office (190/105), so I referred her back to her internist for evaluation. A beta-blocker, a type of blood pressure medication, was prescribed to treat her hypertension. Within a few weeks, her blood pressure returned to normal.

When we saw Nancy back for her next eye examination three months later, she reported "feeling lousy" and "being constantly tired." She also reported being anxious and worrying about her sugars running low. She noted that she used to be able to tell when this was happeniing; she would feel shaky and get sweaty. Now she had few symptoms and found herself checking her sugars frequently just to reassure herself. She also admitted to feeling depressed and not wanting to go to work or visit with friends. She wondered if this was a change in her diabetes, the new medication, or just the winter blues. Despite her significantly improved hypertension, Nancy felt lousy. The beta-blocker was masking her hypoglycemic episodes and contributing to her mild depression. We spoke with her internist, who agreed to change her medication. Nancy is now back to her usual cheerful self.

APPENDIX A

State Agencies for the Visually Impaired

Alabama
Alabama Division of Vocational
Rehabilitation and Crippled
Children Services
2129 East South Blvd.
P.O. Box 11586
Montgomery, AL 36111-0586
(205) 281-8780

Alaska
Alaska Office of
Vocational Rehabilitation
P.O. Box F, Mail Stop 0581
Juneau, AK 99811-0581
(907) 465-2814

Arizona
Arizona State Services for the
Blind and Visually Impaired
4620 North 16 Street, Suite 100
Phoenix, AZ 85016
(602) 255-1850

Arkansas
Arkansas Division of Services
for the Blind
411 Victory Street
P.O. Box 3237
Little Rock, AR 72202
(501) 324-9270

California
California Department of
Rehabilitation
Central Office, 830 K Street Mall
Sacramento, CA 95814
(916) 445-3971

Colorado
Division of Rehabilitation,
Colorado Rehabilitation
Services
1575 Sherman Street
Denver, CO 80203-1714
(303) 866-4390

Connecticut
Connecticut State Board of
Education and Services
for the Blind
170 Ridge Road
Wethersfield, CT 06109
(203) 249-8525

Delaware
Delaware Division for the
Visually Impaired
305 West Eighth Street
Wilmington, DE 19801
(302) 577-333

District of Columbia
District of Columbia
Rehabilitation Services
Administration
Visual Impairment Section
605 G Street, Room 901
Washington, DC 20001
(202) 727-0907

Florida
Division of Blind Services
Florida Department of
Education
2540 Executive Center
Circle West
Tallahassee, FL 32399
(904) 488-1330

Georgia
Georgia Division of
Rehabilitation Services
878 Peachtree Street, NE
Atlanta, GA 30309
(404) 894-6670

Guam
Guam Department of
Vocational Rehabilitation
GCIC Building, 9th Floor
414 West Soledad Avenue
Agana, GU 96910
011 + (671) 472-8806

Hawaii
Hawaii Department of
Human Services, Services for
the Blind Branch
1901 Bachelor Street
Honolulu, HI 96817
(808) 548-7408

Idaho
Idaho Commission
for the Blind
341 West Washington
Boise, ID 83702
(208) 334-3220

Illinois
State of Illinois Department of
Rehabilitation Services
622 East Washington Street
P.O. Box 19429
Springfield, IL 62794-9429
(217) 782-2093

Indiana
Indiana Rehabilitation Services/
Division of Services for the
Blind and Visually Impaired
150 West Market Street
P.O. Box 7083
Indianapolis, IN 46207-7083
(317) 232-1433

Iowa
Iowa Department for the Blind
524 Fourth Street
Des Moines, IA 50309
(515) 281-7999

Kansas
Kansas Division of Services
for the Blind
Biddle Building, 2nd Floor
300 SW Oakley
Topeka, KS 66606
(913) 296-4454

Kentucky
Kentucky Department
for the Blind
427 Versailles Road
Frankfort, KY 40601
(502) 564-4754

Louisiana
Louisiana Rehabilitation
Services
1755 Florida Blvd., 1st Floor
P.O. Box 94371
Baton Rouge, LA 70804-9371
(504) 342-5284

Maine
Maine Bureau of Rehabilitation
Division of the Visually Impaired
35 Anthony Avenue
Augusta, ME 04333
(207) 626-5323

Maryland
Maryland Division of
Vocational Rehabilitation
2301 Argonne Drive
Baltimore, MD 21218
(301) 554-3276

Massachusetts
Massachusetts Commission for
the Blind
88 Kingston Street
Boston, MA 02111
(617) 727-5550

Michigan
Department of Labor/Michigan
Commission for the Blind
201 North Washington Square
P.O. Box 30015
Lansing, MI 48909
(517) 373-2062

Minnesota
Minnesota State Services
for the Blind and Visually
Handicapped
1745 University Avenue West
St. Paul, MN 55104
(612) 642-0500

Mississippi
Department of Human Services
Division of Vocational
Rehabilitation for the Blind
5455 Executive Place
P.O. Box 4872
Jackson, MS 39296-4872
(601) 354-6411

Missouri
Missouri Bureau for the Blind
619 East Capitol Avenue
Jefferson City, MO 65101
(314) 751-4249

Montana
Visual Services Division/
Montana Department of Social
and Rehabilitation Services
111 Sanders
P.O. Box 4210
Helena, MT 59604
(406) 444-2590

Nebraska
Nebraska Division of
Rehabilitation Services
for the Visually Impaired
4600 Valley Road
Lincoln, NE 68510
(402) 471-2891

Nevada
Nevada Bureau of Services to
the Blind, Kinkead Building
505 East King Street, Room 503
Carson City, NV 89710
(702) 687-444

New Hampshire
New Hampshire Division of
Vocational Rehabilitation/
Bureau of Blind Services
78 Regional Drive, Building 2
Concord, NH 03301
(603) 271-3537

New Jersey
New Jersey Commission for the
Blind and Visually Impaired
153 Halsey Street
P.O. Box 47017
Newark, NJ 07101
(973) 648-2111

New Mexico
New Mexico Commission for
the Blind
Pera Building, Room 205
Santa Fe, NM 87503
(505) 827-4479

New York
New York State Commission
for the Blind and Visually
Handicapped
40 North Pearl Street
Albany, NY 12243
(518) 474-6812

North Carolina
North Carolina Department of
Human Resources/Division of
Services for the Blind
309 Ashe Avenue
Raleigh, NC 27606-2102
(919) 733-9822

North Dakota
North Dakota Office of Voca-
tional Rehabilitation
Capitol Building
Bismarck, ND 58505
(701) 224-2907

Ohio
Ohio Rehabilitation Services
Commission Bureau of Services
for the Visually Impaired
400 East Campus View Blvd.
Columbus, OH 43235-4604
(614) 438-1255

Oklahoma

Oklahoma State Office of
Visual Services
2409 North Kelly Street
Oklahoma City, OK 73111
(405) 424-6006

Oregon

Oregon State Commission for
the Blind
535 SE 12th Avenue
Portland, OR 97214
(503) 238-8375

Pennsylvania

Pennsylvania Bureau of
Blindness and Visual Services
Bertelino Bldg., 1st Floor
P.O. Box 2675
Harrisburg, PA 17105
(717) 787-6176

Puerto Rico

Vocational Rehabilitation
Program, Puerto Rico
Department of Social Services
Box 1118
Hato Rey, PR 00919
(809) 725-1792 or
724-7400, ext. 2335

Rhode Island

Rhode Island Services for the
Blind and Visually Impaired
275 Westminster Street
Providence, RI 02903
(401) 277-2300

South Carolina

South Carolina Commission
for the Blind
1430 Confederate Avenue
Columbia, SC 29201
(803) 734-7522

South Dakota

Division of Services to the
Blind and Visually Impaired
South Dakota Department of
Human Services
700 Governors Drive
Pierre, SD 57501-2291
(605) 773-3195

Tennessee

Tennessee Services
for the Blind
Citizens Plaza Bldg., 11th Floor
400 Deadrick Street
Nashville, TN 37248-6200
(615) 741-2095

Texas

Texas Commission for the Blind
Administration Building
4800 North Lamar Blvd.
P.O. Box 12866
Austin, TX 788711
(512) 549-2500

Utah

Utah Division of Services for
the Visually Handicapped
309 East 100 South
Salt Lake City, UT 84111
(801) 533-9393

Vermont
Vermont Division for the Blind
and Visually Impaired
Osgood Building
103 South Main Street
Waterbury, VT 05676
(802) 241-2210

Virginia
Virginia Department for the
Visually Handicapped
397 Azalea Avenue
Richmond, VA 23227
(804) 371-3140

Virgin Islands
Division of Vocational
Rehabilitation
Virgin Islands Department of
Social Welfare
P.O. Box 550, Charlotte Amalie
St. Thomas, VI 00801
(809) 774-0930

Washington
Washington State Department
of Services for the Blind
521 East Legion Way
Mailstop SD-11
Olympic, WA 98504-1422
(206) 586-1224

West Virginia
West Virginia Division of
Vocational Rehabilitation
Blind Adjustment Unit
P.O. Box 1004
Institute, WV 25112
(304) 766-4600

Wisconsin
Wisconsin Division of
Vocational Rehabilitation
Services for the Blind
1 West Wilson Street
Madison, WI 53707
(608) 266-1281

Wyoming
Division of Vocational
Rehabilitation
Wyoming Department of
Employment
1100 Herschler Building
Cheyenne, WY 82002
(307) 777-7385

APPENDIX B

Agencies and Organizations Serving the Blind and Visually Impaired

American Council of the Blind, Inc.
1155 15th Street NW, Suite 20
Washington, DC 20005
(202) 467-5081
1-800-424-8666
(weekday afternoons,
3:00–5:30 EST)

American Diabetes Association National Service Center
1660 Duke Street
Alexandria, VA 22314
(703) 549-1500

American Foundation for the Blind
15 West 16th Street
New York, NY 10011
1-800-232-5463 (hotline)

American Printing House for the Blind
P.O. Box 6085
1839 Frankfort Avenue
Louisville, KY 40206
(502) 895-2405

Association for Education and Rehabilitation of the Blind and Visually Impaired
206 North Washington Street, Suite 320
Alexandria, VA 22314
(703) 548-1884

Association for Macular Diseases
210 East 64th Street
New York, NY 10021
(212) 605-3719

Association of Radio Reading Services
University of Southern Florida
WRB 209
Tampa, Florida 33620
(813) 974-4193

Blinded Veterans Association
477 H Street NW
Washington, DC 20001
(202) 371-8880
1-800-699-7079

Blind Outdoor Leisure Development
St. Mary's Church
533 East Main Street
Aspen, CO 81611
(303) 925-8922

Carroll Center for the Blind
700 Centre Street
Newton, MA 02158
(617) 969-6200

Center for Independent Living
817 Broadway, 11th Floor
New York, NY 10003
(212) 477-3800

Corneal Dystrophy Foundation
1926 Hidden Creek Drive
Kingwood, TX 77339
(713) 358-4227

The Foundation Fighting Blindness
Executive Plaza 1, Suite 800
11350 McCormick Road
Hunt Valley, MD 21031-1014
1-800-683-5555
1-800-683-5551 TDD

Foundation for Glaucoma Research
490 Post Street, Suite 830
San Francisco, CA 94102
(415) 986-3162

Helen Keller National Center for Deaf-Blind Youths and Adults
111 Middle Neck Road
Sands Point, NY 11050
(516) 944-8900 (Voice & TDD)

Hill Burton Program (Uncompensated Services)
Health Resources and Services Administration
5600 Fishers Lane, Room 11-19
Rockville, MD 20857

IBM National Support Center for Persons with Disabilities
P.O. Box 2150
Atlanta, GA 30301-2150
1-800-426-2133

International Association of Lions Clubs (Lions Clubs International)
300 22nd Street
Oak Brook, IL 60521-8842
(708) 571-5466

International Institute for Visually Impaired (0–7)
1975 Rutgers Circle
East Lansing, MI 48823

Library of Congress National Library Service for the Blind and Physically Handicapped
1291 Taylor Street, NW
Washington, DC 20542
1-800-424-9100

Lions' Club International
330 22nd Street
Oakbrook, IL 60521-8842
(708) 571-5466

March of Dimes Birth Defects Foundation
1275 Mamaroneck Avenue
White Planes, NY 10605
(914) 428-7100

Mission Cataract USA
6766 N Cedar Avenue, Suite 212
Fresno, CA 93710
1-800-343-7265

Myasthenia Gravis Foundation
61 Gramercy Park North
New York, NY 10010
(212) 533-7005

National Accreditation Council for Agencies Serving the Blind and Visually Handicapped
232 Madison Avenue, Suite 907
New York, NY 10016
(212) 779-8080

National Association for Parents of the Visually Impaired, Inc.
2180 Linway Drive
Beloit, WI 53511
1-800-562-6265

National Association for Visually Handicapped
22 West 21st Street
New York, NY 10010
(212) 889-3141

National Diabetes Information Clearinghouse (NDIC)
One Information Way
Bethesda, MD 20892-3560
(301) 654-3327

National Elder Care Institute of Health Promotion
601 E Street NW, 5th Floor
Washington, DC 20049
(202) 434-2200

National Eye Institute
National Institutes of Health
Box 20/20, Bldg. 31, Room 6A32
Bethesda, MD 20892
(301) 496-5248

National Federation of the Blind
1800 Johnson Street
Baltimore, MD 21230
(301) 659-9314

National Institute on Aging Information Center
P.O. Box 8057
Gaithersburg, MD 20898-8057
1-800-222-2225

National Multiple Sclerosis Society
205 East 42nd Street, 3rd Floor
New York, NY 10017
(212) 986-3240

National Rehabilitation Information Center (NARIC)
8455 Colesville Road, Suite 935
Silver Springs, MD 20910
1-800-346-2742

National Retinitis Pigmentosa Foundation, Inc.
1401 Mt. Royal Avenue,
4th Floor
Baltimore, MD 21217
1-800-638-2300
(301) 225-9409 TDD

National Society to Prevent Blindness
500 East Remington Road
Schaumberg, IL 60173
1-800-331-2020

Office of Disease Prevention and Health Promotion (ODPHP), National Health Information Center
P.O. Box 1133
Washington, DC 20013-1133
1-800-336-4797

Office of Minority Health Resource Center
P.O. Box 37337
Washington DC 20013-7337
1-800-444-6472

Prevent Blindness America
Center for Sight
500 East Remington Road
Schaumburg, IL 60173-4557
1-800-331-2020

Recording for the Blind
20 Roszel Road
Princeton, NJ 08540
(609) 452-0606

Salvation Army Divisional Headquarters
120 West 14th Street
New York, NY 10011
(212) 337-7200

Talking Books: National Library Service for the Blind and Visually Handicapped
Library of Congress
Washington, DC 20540
1-800-424-9100

APPENDIX C

Resources

GENERAL DIABETES

American Academy of Ophthalmology
Public Information Program
P.O. Box 7424
San Francisco, CA 94120-7424
(415) 561-8520
Diabetic Retinopathy
Referral Program
1-800-628-6733
E-mail: ips@aao.org
Membership organization for ophthalmologists; referral program for diabetic eye disease screening; provides brochures and eye fact sheets, educational materials

American Association of Diabetes Educators
444 North Michigan Avenue,
Suite 1240
Chicago, IL 60611

1-800-832-6874
(312) 644-2233
http://www.AADEnet.org

American Diabetes Association
1660 Duke Street
Alexandria, VA 22314
1-800-232-3472
1-800-Diabetes
(703) 549-1500
http://www.diabetes.org

Canadian Diabetes Association
78 Bond Street
Toronto, Ontario M5B 2J8
Canada

Centers for Disease Control and Prevention (CDC)
Division of Diabetes Translation
National Center for Chronic
Disease, Prevention, and Health
Promotion

TISB Mail Stop K-13
4770 Buford Highway NE
Atlanta, GA 30341-3724
(770) 488-5080
Fax: (770) 488-5969
http://www.cdc.gov

Endocrine Society
4350 East West Highway,
Suite 500
Bethesda, MD 20814-4410
(301) 941-0200
Fax: (301) 941-0259
http://www.endo-society.org
E-mail: endostaff@endo-
society.org

Indian Health Service (IHS)
Diabetic Program,
Headquarters West
5300 Homestead Road, NE
Albuquerque, NM 87110
(505) 837-4182
Fax: (505) 437-4188
*Diabetes resources available;
general information; training
programs; audiovisual learning
tools*

**International Diabetes
Federation**
1 rue Defacqz
B-1000
Brussels, Belgium
32-2/538-5511
Fax: 32-2-538-5114
E-mail: idf@idf.org
http://www.idf.org
*Provides grants for research,
education, courses, inter-
national training; provides*

*up-to-date information about
diabetes and essential
research; exchange network;
IDF newsletter*

Joslin Diabetes Center
One Joslin Place
Boston, MA 02215
(617) 732-2695
http://www.joslin.harvard.edu
*Medical treatment for all
people with diabetes; research
related to all facets of diabetes;
medical education*

National Eye Institute
E-mail: 2020@b31.nei.nih.gov
http://www.nei.nih.gov
*Conducts cutting-edge eye
research; keeps the public
abreast of research; promotes
public and private awareness of
importance of early diagnosis
and treatment of diabetic eye
disease; provides materials*

**National Institute of
Diabetes and Digestive and
Kidney Diseases**
http://www.niddk.nih.gov
*Diabetes research institute
branch of U.S. National
Institutes of Health; information on diabetic complications, diabetic statistics, blood
glucose control, professional
and voluntary diabetes
organizations*

Veteran's Health Administration
Diabetes Program, Headquarters
810 Vermont Avenue, NW
Washington, DC 20420
(202) 273-8490
Fax: (202) 273-9142

PEDIATRICS

Children with Diabetes
http://www.castleweb.com

International Society for Pediatric and Adolescent Diabetes (ISPAD)
c/o New England Diabetes and
Endocrinology Center
40 Second Avenue, Suite 170
Waltham, MA 02154-1132
(617) 890-3610
Fax: (617) 890-3612

Juvenile Diabetes Foundation International
120 Wall Street, 19th Floor
New York, NY 10005-4001
(212) 785-9500
1-800-533-2873
1-800-JDF-CURE
http://www.jdfcure.com
Information about JDF and local chapters; general diabetes information; research news; government relations information; selected articles from Countdown

Juvenile Diabetes Foundation Canada
89 Granton Drive
Richmond Hill, Ontario
Canada L4B 2N5
(905) 889-4171

(See also **Lighthouse Center for Education**)

INFORMATION ABOUT VISUAL IMPAIRMENTS

American Council of the Blind
1155 15th Street NW, Suite 720
Washington, DC 20005
(202) 467-5081
http://www.acb.org
Membership organization ($25); provides resource lists, monthly magazine (free) in Braille, large print, or cassette, college scholarships, rehabilitation training, talking books

American Foundation for the Blind
11 Penn Plaza, Suite 300
New York, NY 10001
Excellent public education materials; free public education materials catalog; offers various publications

Blinded Veteran's Association (BVA)
Publishes BVA bulletin; scholarship programs

Council of Citizens with Low Vision (CCLVI)
c/o Teresa Blessing
6511 26th Street West
Bradenton, FL 34207
1-800-733-2258
Membership organization; offers scholarships for students majoring in low-vison rehabilitation; newsletter; low-vision resources

Equal Opportunity Publications, Inc.
150 Motor Parkway, Suite 420
Hauppauge, NY 11788-5145
Quarterly publication, $10; interview strategies for people with and without disabilities

Glaucoma Research Foundation
490 Post Street, Suite 830
San Francisco, CA 94102
1-800-826-6693
(415) 986-3162
(415) 986-3763
glaucoma@itsa.ucsf.edu
Sponsors and conducts research; provides comprehensive patient education materials and support services; monthly newsletter

Leader Dogs for the Blind
Rochester Leader Dog School
(313) 651-9011
(248) 651-3713 (TTY)

The Lighthouse, Inc.
111 East 59th Street
New York, NY 10022
1-800-334-5497
(212) 821-9713 TDD
http://www.lighthouse.org
E-mail: csussman@lighthouse.org
Free copy of "Introduction to Adaptive Computer Technology" and "Shared Solutions to Adaptive Living":
jjenkins@lighthouse.org
Information and resource service on eye conditions and visual impairment for all ages; assists with every aspect of low vision and provides invaluable resource information on low-vision devices, rehabilitation, aging, children with visual impairment, and recommendations of low-vision specialists throughout the country; technical consultation; catalog of low-vision aids

National Association for Visually Handicapped (NAVH)
22 West 21st Street, 6th Floor
New York, NY 10010
(212) 889-3141
http://www.NAVH.org
Leading library of large-print materials for members; large-print loan libraries; information packet; visual aids; emotional and peer support, senior outreach programs

National Federation of the Blind Diabetics Division (NFB)
811 Cherry Street, Suite 306
Columbia, MO 65201
(314) 875-8911

National Federation of the Blind (NFB)
1800 Johnson Street
Baltimore, MD 21230
(410) 659-9314
Blind and sighted members; national magazine, literature in large print, Braille, cassette, and talking books; referral and job services

National Library Service for the Blind and Physically Handicapped
Library of Congress
1291 Taylor Street, NW
Washington, DC 20542
1-800-424-8567
Offers publications in Braille, large-print, and recorded form, free of charge to those with visual impairments; publishes free and informative fact sheets, reference circulars, and bibliographies on many topics; request brochure and application

Resources for Rehabilitation
33 Bedford Street, Suite 19A
Lexington, MA 02173
(617) 862-6455
(617) 861-7517
Large-print directories, large-print resource lists

Vision Foundation, Inc.
818 Mt. Auburn Street
Watertown, MA 02172
Publishes "vision resource list" with roughly 150 catalogs, brochures, organizations, etc.; check which items you want (large print, Braille, cassette); information on those items will be mailed

INFORMATION FOR CHILDREN WITH VISUAL IMPAIRMENTS

The Institute for Families with Blind Children
Mail Stop #111
P.O. Box 54700
Los Angeles, CA 90054-0700
(213) 669-4649
Quarterly newsletter free to parents and professionals; counseling and support services

The Lighthouse National Center for Vision and Child Development
111 East 59th Street
New York, NY 10022
1-800-334-5497
(212) 821-9713 TDD

http://www.lighthouse.org
*Information on visual impair-
ment in kids of all ages;
resources, education and
printed materials; consultation available*

National Association for Parents of the Visually Impaired
*Support for children with
visual impairments*

SERVICES FOR PERSONS WITH VISUAL IMPAIRMENTS

Financial Help and Services

Legal services: May be
offered at a discount or free of
charge to those in financial
need; contact your local bar
association or the Yellow
Pages for Legal Clinics for
the Disabled

Local banks: They may accept
large-print checks or may offer
bank by phone services; if
large-print checks are unavail-
able locally, you may wish to
order them from:

Guideline Checks
Deluxe Check Printing Co.
4 Industrial Blvd.
Paoli, PA 19301
(620) 647-7667

Phone companies: Free
directory assistance services
available from:

AT&T ACLDSC
P.O. Box 45006
Dallas, TX 75245-0006
1-800-872-3883
Contact your local phone car-
rier to inquire about free directory assistance in your area

**Social Security Administra-
tion:** Individuals may qualify
for Social Security Disability
Insurance or Supplemental
Security Income or both—
if so, they may be eligible for
Medicare or Medicaid; contact
local Social Security Office to
explore eligibility

Utility companies: Offer bills
in large print, Braille, or may
even be willing to read your bill
over the phone; inquire

Transportation Agencies

Airlines and cruise ships:
Special assistance when
requested

Amtrak: Reduced fares, special assistance when requested

**Local transportation
authorities:** May offer
reduced-fare programs

National Library Service for the Blind: "Information for Handicapped Travelers" reference circular

Private bus lines: Greyhound and Trailways allow a companion to travel with a disabled person to provide assistance for the price of a single adult fare

Recreation and Cultural Attractions

Parks and museums: Offer discounts; always ask

National Park Service: Free Golden Access PassPort for those receiving federal benefits; passport gives free admission to national parks, discounts on camping and activities

Educational Services

American Printing House for the Blind
1839 Frankfort Avenue
P.O. Box 6085
Louisville, KY 40206
1-800-223-1839
Offers large-print, Braille, and recorded texts, various educational materials; offers Newsweek *and* Reader's Digest *on cassette free to users of the library for the blind and dyslexic*

Hadley School for the Blind
700 Elm Street
P.O. Box 299
Winnetka, IL 60093
Free correspondence courses covering many subjects

Recordings for the Blind and Dyslexic
20 Roszel Road
Princeton, NJ 08540
1-800-221-4792
Recorded texts for students; recorded professional and technical materials for professionals in many fields

Leisure Activities

Disabled Sports USA
451 Hungerford Drive,
Suite 100
Rockville, MD 20850
(301) 393-7505

International Diabetic Athletes Association
1647-B West Bethany Home Road
Phoenix, AZ 85015
1-800-898-IDAA
(602) 433-2113
Fax: (602) 433-9331
http://www.getnet.com
E-mail: idaa@getnet.com
Network of athletes with diabetes; quarterly newsletter The Challenge

**U.S. Association of
Blind Athletes**
33 N. Institute Street
West Hall
Colorado Springs, CO 80903
(719) 630-0422

Very Special Arts
1300 Connecticut Avenue,
Suite 700
Washington, DC 20036
(202) 628-2800
(202) 737-0645 TDD
*U.S. coordinating agency of
arts programs for those with
disabilities*

PRODUCTS FOR THOSE WITH VISUAL IMPAIRMENTS

The following resources provide
helpful products for home,
leisure, and work, as well as
toys and games:

Ann Morris Enterprises, Inc.
890 Fams Court
East Meadow, NY 11554
1-800-454-3175

Independent Living Aids, Inc.
27 East Mall
Plainview, NY 11803
1-800-537-2118
(516) 752-8080
Fax: (516) 752-3135

LS&S Group, Inc.
Box 673
Northbrook, IL 60065
1-800-468-4789

Maxi Aids
42 Executive Blvd.
Box 3209
Farmingdale, NY 11735
1-800-468-4789

**National Association for
Visually Handicapped**
22 West 21st Street, 6th Floor
New York, NY 10010
(212) 889-3141
http://www.NAVH.org
*Provides counseling in testing,
use, and purchase of visual
aids and special illumination
devices*

Large-Print Materials

American Bible Society
1865 Broadway
New York, NY 10023
(212) 408-1200

Bible Alliance, Inc.
P.O. Box 621
Bradenton, FL 34206
(941) 748-3031
Fax: (941) 748-2625
*Recorded scriptures in forty
languages on cassettes; tapes
free to blind, visually
impaired, partially sighted
(verification of handicap
required); free demonstration
sets for patient resource
centers*

Blindskills, Inc.
P.O. Box 5181
Salem, OR 97304-0181
(503) 581-4224
Fax: (503) 581-0178
*Quarterly magazines, large
print, Braille, and 4-track
cassettes*

Books on Tape, Inc.
P.O. Box 7900
Newport Beach, CA 92658-7900
1-800-626-3333
*Provides a rental program of
full-length books from classics
to best-sellers*

Braille Circulation Library
2700 Stuart Avenue
Richmond, VA 23220-3305
(804) 359-3743
Fax: (804) 359-4777
*Provides Braille and talking
book tapes, cassettes, and large-
print materials*

Chivers of North America
P.O. Box 1450
Hampton, NH 03843-1450
1-800-621-0182
*Audiobooks, unabridged
novels, particularly by
British authors*

**Doubleday Large Print
Home Center**
Membership Service Center
6550 East 30th Street
Box 6325
Indianapolis, IN 46206
(317) 541-8920

*Membership includes literary
information and discounted
large-print best-seller books,
cassettes, music tapes, and
videos*

GK Hall and Co.
P.O. Box 159
Thorndike, ME 04986
1-800-223-6121
(207) 948-2962
Fax: 1-800-558-4674
Direct sale of large-print books

**John Milton Society
for the Blind**
475 Riverside Drive, Room 455
New York, NY 10115
(212) 870-3336
Fax: (212) 870-3229
*Free large-print type, directory
of resources, and Christian
literature in Braille, 4-track,
cassettes*

Large Print Literary Reader
Dept. W
955 Massachusetts Avenue #105
Cambridge, MA 02139
(617) 354-5446
E-mail: csz112a@prodigy.com
*Essays, fiction, and history in
large print*

Local libraries (see Yellow
Page directories)
(see **National Library
Service for the Blind**)

New York Times Mail Subscriptions
P.O. Box 3009
South Hackensack, NJ 07606
1-800-631-2580

New York Times Large Print Weekly
229 West 43rd Street
New York, NY 10036
1-800-631-2580
(212) 556-1734
Large-type weekly subscription

Random House
400 Hahn Road
Westminster, MD 21157
1-800-726-0600

Reader's Digest Association
Large-Type Publications
Box 241
Mount Morris, IL 61054
1-800-877-5293
(815) 734-6963
Reader's Digest, *condensed books*, Great Bibliographies, *and the Bible*

Thorndike Press
P.O. Box 159
Thorndike, ME 04986
1-800-223-6121
(207) 948-2762
Fax: 1-800-558-4676
Direct sale of large-print books

Ulverscroft Large Print (USA), Inc.
P.O. Box 1230
West Seneca, NY 14224-1230
1-800-955-9059
(716) 674-4270
(716) 674-4195

World at Large, Inc.
1689 46th Street
Brooklyn, NY 11204
1-800-285-2743
(718) 972-4000
Fax: (718) 972-9400
Biweekly large-print newspaper which prints articles from magazines such as US News and World Report, Time, *and* The Monitor

Lighting Products

Available through low-vision product catalogs, local lighting stores, office supply, or department stores.

Big Eye Lamp, Inc.
133 Yellowbrook Road
Farmingdale, NJ 07727
1-800-242-8311

Comfort Plus High-Intensity Lighting and Reading Stands
Bob Cope
1136 Gibbsboro Road
Kirkwood, NJ 08043
(609) 784-6444

Dazor Manufacturing Corp.
4483 Duncan Avenue
St. Louis, MO 63110
1-800-345-9103

Goodwin Manufacturing Co.
P.O. Box 378
241 Main Street
Luck, WI 54853
1-800-282-5267

Luxo Lamp Corp.
36 Midland Avenue
Port Chester, NY 10573
1-800-222-5896

Radio Reading Service

In Touch Networks
322 West 48th Street
New York, NY 10036
(212) 769-6270
*Radio reading service
available in thirty-five states
via satellite*

Recorded Materials

Choice Magazine Listening
85 Channel Drive
Port Washington, NY 11050
(516) 883-8280
Fax: (516) 944-6849
*Selected magazines, stories,
and poetry on cassette;
subscriptions are free*

**Christian Record
Services, Inc.**
4444 South 52nd Street
P.O. Box 6097
Lincoln, NE 68506

(402) 488-0981
Fax: (402) 488-7582
(402) 488-1902 TDD
*Provides free Christian publi-
cations and programs for persons with visual or hearing
impairments; includes magazines in Braille, large print,
and cassette tape; lending
library; Bible correspondence
school; national camps for
blind children*

**Matilda Ziegler Magazine
for the Blind**
80 8th Avenue
Room 1304
New York, NY 10011
(212) 242-0263

Descriptive Video Service

WGBH
125 Western Avenue
Boston, MA 02134
(617) 492-2777, ext 3490
*Action in specific programs
is described during gaps in
dialogue*

Religious Materials

See National Library Service
for the Blind circular, "Bibles,
Other Scriptures, Liturgies, and
Hymnals in Special Media."
Many other sources of such
materials are listed here:

Christian Association for Rehabilitation and Education Ministries (CARE)
P.O. Box 1830
Starkville, MS 39760
(601) 323-4999
Serves as an information and referral clearinghouse for religious materials and varied services and organizations

Jewish Braille Institute of America
110 East 30th Street
New York, NY 10016
(212) 889-2525
Large print, talking book, and Braille library of Jewish materials

SOFTWARE PRODUCTS FOR DIABETES MANAGEMENT

Balance PC Diabetes Software
Medilife, Inc.
1-888-656-5656
Compatible glucometer: all meters able to store data
Estimated cost: $59.95

CAMIT Diabetes Management Software
Cascade Medical, Inc.
1-800-525-6718
Compatible glucometer: Accu-Chek Advantage, Accu-Chek Easy, Accu-Chek Instant DM, Accu-Chek III, and Merlin Electronic Logbook
Estimated cost: $69.99

Check Link Diabetes Care Software
Cascade Medical, Inc.
1-800-525-6718
Compatible glucometer:
Checkmate Plus
Estimated cost: $39.95

Diabetic Mentor
Vigora
1-800-743-5680
Compatible glucometer: One Touch II, One Touch Profile
Estimated cost: $49.95

In Touch Diabetes Management Software
Lifescan, Inc.
1-800-227-8862
Compatible glucometer: One Touch II, One Touch Profile
Estimated cost: $89.99

Level Healthware
1-800-682-9375
Compatible glucometer: One Touch II, One Touch Profile
Estimated cost: $89.99

Mellitus Manager
MetaMedix, Inc.
1-800-455-4105
Compatible glucometer: One Touch II, One Touch Profile, Accu-Chek Advantage, Accu-Chek Profile, Accu-Chek Easy, MediSense 2, Precision QID
Estimated cost: $79.95

Precision Link
MediSense
1-800-527-3339
Compatible glucometer: Precision QID, MediSense 2
Estimated cost: $139.95

Software Products for Nutritional Diabetic Management

Meals 'n' Carbs
Diabetes Educators, Inc.
P.O. Box 1393
Bryn Mawr, PA 19010-7393
or
3930 NE 2nd Avenue, Suite 204
Miami, FL 33137
(305) 576-0444
Fax: (305) 576-0509
CD-ROM for PC/Macintosh that teaches carbohydrate counting, nutrition, and the basics of diabetes; interactive, voice; great for kids

ADAPTIVE TECHNOLOGY

Local agencies and organizations for the visually impaired may offer information, demonstrations, evaluations, financial assistance, and other help for those interested in adaptive technology for people with visual impairments. Adaptive technology centers, where an individual can be evaluated to determine the appropriate computer access solution, may be available locally.

American Printing House for the Blind
1839 Frankfort Avenue
P.O. Box 6085
Louisville, KY 40206
1-800-223-1839
Makers of "The Big Picture," a handheld camera that turns a TV into a closed circuit television (CCTV)

CTech
P.O. Box 30
2 North William Street
Pearl River, NY 10965-9998
1-800-228-7798
Varied computer products; closed circuit televisions; rental program available; used CCTVs available

Human Ware, Inc.
6245 King Road
Loomis, CA 95650
1-800-722-3393

IBM Independence Series Information Center
P.O. Box 1328
Boca Raton, FL 34429-1328
1-800-426-4832

Innovations
5921 S. Middlefield Rd., Suite 102
Littleton, CO 80123-2877
1-800-854-6554
(303) 797-6554
Fax: (303) 727-4940
E-mail:
magnicam@magnicam.com
http://www.magnicam.com/magnicam/

*Manufacturer of Magni-Cam™,
a handheld camera that turns
a TV into a closed circuit
television; also available in
portable form*

(See also **National
Association for Visually
Handicapped**)

National Technology Center
American Foundation
for the Blind
11 Penn Plaza, Suite 300
New York, NY 10001
(212) 502-7600

Optelec
6 Liberty Way
P.O. Box 729
Westford, MA 01886
1-800-828-1056
*Varied computer products,
closed circuit televisions*

TeleSensory
455 North Beranardo Avenue
Mountain View, CA 94043
1-800-804-8004
*Varied computer products,
closed circuit televisions*

APPENDIX D

Medication Assistance Programs for the Needy

General Guidelines

❖ Patients must be considered "medically needy" by a physician

❖ Patients must not be eligible for third-party coverage (Medicare, Medicaid, private insurance)

❖ Pharmaceutical company information forms must be completed and signed by a physician

❖ Renewal of paperwork after prescribed time period

❖ Inclusion of original prescription(s)

❖ Medications are shipped to the ophthalmologist's office for dispersal

❖ Each company reserves the right to discontinue or modify its program at any time

❖ For other systemic medications needed, see "Directory of Pharmaceutical Manufacturers Programs"

ALCON LABORATORIES

Program Name: Alcon Needy Assistance Program
Phone: 1-800-451-3937
Address: Manager, Physician Services
Alcon Laboratories, Inc.
6201 South Freeway
Fort Worth, TX 76134-2099

Eligibility:	Deemed medically needy by physician (practicing eye care specialist)
	Ineligible for third-party reimbursement
	Private patient
Requirements:	Written request
Include:	Doctor's name, original signature, state license number, patient's name, quantity and concentration of each medication requested
Medications:	Betoptic S 0.25% (2 ea., 15 ml)
	Betoptic 0.50% (2 ea., 15 ml)
	Isopto Carpine 1% (3 ea., 15 ml), 2%, 3%, 4%, 6% (3 ea., 30 ml)
	Isopto Carbachol 0.75% (3 ea., 15 ml), 1.5%, 3% (3 ea., 30 ml)
	Epinal 0.5%,1% (2 ea., 7.5 ml)
	Iopidine 0.5% (2 ea., 10 ml)
	Glaucon 1%, 2% (2 ea., 10 ml)
	PE 1%, 2%, 3%, 4%, 6% Pilocarpine with 1% epinephrine (3 ea., 15 ml)
	Pilopine HS 4% (2 ea., 4.0 gm tubes)

ALLERGAN

Program:	Allergan Patient Assistance Program
Phone:	1-800-347-4500, ext 7791
	(714) 752-4500
Address:	2525 DuPont Drive
	P.O. Box 19534
	Irvine, CA 92612
Eligibility:	Deemed medically indigent by physician. Ineligible for third-party reimbursement. Patient's annual household income must not exceed $12,000 for one- or two-person household or $19,000 for three or more persons.
Requirements:	1. Complete Allergan Information form, *or*
	2. Send the following information on professional letter stationery: Date of request, physician name and address, active state license or DEA number,

Medications:

patient name, specific Allergan product (strength and size), physician's original signature

3. Include dosing frequency with all artificial tear products

Betagan 0.25% (4 ea., 10 ml)

Betagan 0.5% (3 ea., 15 ml)

Pilagan 1%, 2%, 4% (6 ea., 15 ml)

Propine (3 ea., 15 ml)

Epifrin 0.5%, 1%, 2% (3 ea., 15 ml)

Erygel 2%

Elimite 5%

OTC tears: Refresh (30 CT.), Celluvisc (30CT.), Refresh Plus (30 CT.), Refresh PM (3.5G), Tears Plus (½ oz), Lacri-Lube (3.5G)

Duration:

Six-month supply

At the end of six months, paperwork needs to be resubmitted

Contact:

Joan Brewster

ALZA PHARMACEUTICALS

Program Name: c/o Customer Service

Phone: 1-800-227-9953 within U.S.

(415) 962-4149 outside U.S.

(415) 494-5000

Fax: (415) 962-4212 or (415) 962-4141

Address: 950 Page Mill Road

P.O. Box 10950

Palo Alto, CA 94303-0802

Eligibility: Deemed medically needy by physician

Ineligible for third-party reimbursement

Requirements: Completion of information form

Medications: Ocusert Pilo-20

Ocusert Pilo-40

Turnover: UPS shipped—five to seven business days

Refill: Quantity limited to three-month supply

Other Meds: Progestasert, Testoderm Testosterone

ASTRA PHARMACEUTICALS

Program Name:	F.A.I.R.
Phone:	1-800-488-FAIR (3247)
Fax:	(703) 706-5925
Address:	1101 King Street, Suite 600
	Alexandria, VA 22314
Eligibility:	Deemed medically needy by physician
	Ineligible for third-party reimbursement
	Patient must have either CMV retinitis or Acyclovir-resistant Herpes Simplex Virus (HSV) 1 or 2
Requirements:	Complete initial form (patient name, date of birth, diagnosis)
	Signed prescription by a physician
	Medication sent to physician's office each month
	Contact by phone or fax each month for monthly request
Medication:	Foscavir
Recommendations:	Call a request in by phone
	Application sent to physician within twenty-four hours
	F.A.I.R analyzes patient's insurance coverage options
	Turnover is as fast as forty-eight hours
Refill:	Every six months
Contact:	None; Staff of six analysts

CHIRON VISION

Program Name:	None
Phone:	1-800-531-2020
Address:	9342 Jeronimo Road
	Irvine, CA 92718
Requirements:	Hospital and physician must waive their surgical fees
Medications:	Vitrasert
Contact:	Gregory Sanchez

CIBA VISION OPHTHALMICS

Program Name:	Ciba Vision Ophthalmics Patient Assistance Program
Phone:	(770) 418-4008
Address:	11460 Johns Creek Parkway
	Duluth, GA 30155
Eligibility:	Deemed medically needy by physician
	Ineligible for third-party reimbursement
Requirements:	Complete the Ciba Visions Information Form which includes: date of request, physician name and address, state license number or DEA number, patient name, specific CIBA Vision ophthalmic product requested (strength and size), physician's original signature, prescription
Medications:	AquaSite MD and SDU
	Betimol 0.25%, 0.50%
	E-Pilo 1%, 2%, 4%, 6%
	Eyescrubs Premoistened Pads
	HypoTears
	HypoTears Ointment
	HypoTears PF
	Livostin
	Neptazane 25mg, 50mg
	Pilocar 1%, 2%, 4%, 6%
	Vasocon-A
	Voltaren
Duration:	Six months
Contact:	Susan Szecsey, Program Coordinator
Refill:	Reapply after six months

ESCALON

Program Name:	Case-by-case basis
Phone:	1-800-486-4848
Address:	182 Tamarack Circle
	Skillman, NJ 08558
Eligibility:	Deemed medically needy by physician
	Ineligible for third-party reimbursement
Medications:	Adapto Sil 5000 (Silicone oil)
Contact:	Shawn Mullen

GENENTECH, INC.

Program Name:	Genentech Reimbursement Information Program
Phone:	1-800-879-4747
Address:	Mailstop #99
	c/o Genentech
	460 Point San Bruno Blvd.
	South San Francisco, CA 94080
Eligibility:	Deemed medically needy by physician
	Gross family income of $25,000 or less
	Uninsured
Requirements:	Patients must provide detailed information to ensure the company that they are uninsured and cannot afford the medication
Medication:	TPA, tissue plasminogen activator
Process:	Company provides replacement product to hospital

GLAXO WELLCOME

Program Name:	GlaxoWellcome Patient Assistance Program
Phone:	1-800-722-9294
Address:	P.O. Box 52185
	Phoenix, AZ 85072-9711
Eligibility:	First three months—anyone the physician deems cannot afford medications
Requirements:	Enroll a patient over the phone or complete enrollment paperwork. If enrolled over the phone, complete enrollment paperwork within thirty days. Patient receives a prescription benefits card to use at the pharmacy of choice. A $5 copayment may be required with all medications.
Medications:	Viroptic 1%
	Cortisporin Ointment
	Cortisporin Drops
	Polysporin Ointment
	Neosporin Ointment
	Neosporin Drops
Other Meds (with ophthalmic use):	Daraprim (pyrimethamine), Epivir (lamivudine), Imitrex (sumatriptan succinate), Imuran (azathioprine), Myleran (busulfan), Proloprim

	(trimethoprim), Retrovir (zidovudine), Septra (sulfamethoxazole-trimethoprim), Valtrex (valacyclovir), Wellcovorin (leucovorin calcium), Zovirax (acyclovir)
Other Meds:	Aclovate, Alkeran, Beclovent, Beconase, Beconase AQ, Ceftin, Cortisporin Otic, Cutivate, Emgel, Flonase, Kemadrin, Lamictal, Lanoxicaps, Lanoxin, Mepron, Navelbine, Oxistat, Pediotic Suspension, Purinethol, Semprex-D, Serevent, Temovate, Thioguanine, Trandate, Ventolin, Wellbutrin, Zantac, Zofran, Zyloprim
Refill:	After three-month period, patient must demonstrate income eligibility by submitting a payment stub

LEDERLE LABORATORIES (see also WYETH AYERST)

Phone:	1-800-526-7870
	1-800-568-9938
Fax:	(201) 831-4484
Address:	American Cyanamid, Inc.
	One Cyanamid Plaza
	Wayne, NJ 07470
Requirements:	Physician request
Eligibility:	Ineligible for third-party payment
	Financially indigent
Medications:	Diamox

MERCK AND CO., INC.

Address:	P.O. Box 4
	West Point, PA 19486-0004
Phone:	1-800-994-2111 (computer based)
	Physician will need DEA number
Program Name:	Merck Patient Assistance Program (PAT)
Requirements:	Obtain enrollment envelopes and complete all parts
	Enclose original prescription(s)—up to three per envelope
	Physician and patient signature required
Medications:	Chibroxin
	Lacrisert

Decadron (available in 1998)
Timoptic XE
Timoptic 0.25%, 0.50%
Trusopt 2%
Humosol

Turnover:	Two weeks
Refill:	Three-month supply
	Reapply every three months
Other:	Duplications of forms not accepted

NORD—NATIONAL ORGANIZATION FOR RARE DISORDERS

Program Name:	Physician Services—BOTOX Assistance Program
Phone:	1-800-999-NORD
Address:	P.O. Box 8923
	New Fairfield, CT 06812-8923
Medication:	BOTOX (Allergan)
Eligibility:	Deemed medically needy by physician
	Ineligible for third-party reimbursement
	No child under age twelve
Requirement:	Completion of form by physician and patient
	Patient form includes multiple questions aimed at determining monthly disposable income
	Physician may not charge a fee for injection
Refill:	Every one year
Contact:	Indira Kavirajan
Other Meds:	Sandostatin, Parlodel, Eldepryl, Sandoglobulin, Sandimmune, Neoral, Clozaril

OCUSOFT

Phone:	1-800-233-5469
Address:	5311 Avenue North
	P.O. Box 429
	Rosenburg, TX 77471
Eligibility:	Deemed medically needy by physician
Medication:	Lid scrubs
Contact:	Rosemary Martinez, Vice President of Sales Operations

OTSUKA

Program Name:	Indigent Care Program
Phone:	1-800-562-3974, ext 2143
Address:	2440 Research Blvd.
	Rockville, MD 20850
Eligibility:	Deemed medically needy by physician
	Ineligible for third-party reimbursement
Requirements:	Original prescription signed by physician
	Three-month supply sent
Medications:	Ocupress 1%
Refill:	Every three months
Turnover:	Two months
Contact:	Karen Miller

PFIZER

Program Name:	Pfizer Prescription Assistance Program
Phone:	(212) 573-3954
	1-800-646-4455
Address:	P.O. Box 25457
	Alexandria, VA 22313-5457
Eligibility:	Less than $12,000 for individual; less than $15,000 for family of four
	Ineligible for third-party reimbursement
Requirements:	A letter written on office stationery stating the patient is indigent and ineligible for insurance covering pharmaceuticals
	Original prescription
Medications:	Visine
Other Meds:	Any medication manufactured by Pfizer except birth control pills and narcotics
Turnover:	Three to four weeks after letter received
Refill:	Every three months (repeat letter and prescription)

STORZ (see WYETH-AYERST)

SYNTEX LABS

Program Name:	Roche Syntex Medical Needs Program
Phone:	1-800-285-4484
	1-800-444-4200 (Cytovene medical info line)
	1-800-526-6367 (Emergency line)
	1-800-822-8255
Address:	1100 New York Avenue NW, Suite 200
	East Washington, DC 20005-3934
Eligibility:	Immunosuppressed patient with CMV retinitis
	Ineligible for third-party reimbursement
	Financially indigent
Requirements:	Syntex analyzes each patient's financial situation case by case
	Encourages phone enrollment
	Requests a completed application
	Requires original physician signature on application
	Forty-five-day supply sent to physician's office
Medications:	Cytovene tablets
	Cytovene IV
Turnover:	Three to five working days after application complete
Refill:	Reenroll every fourth shipment
Other Meds:	Naprosyn, Anaprox, Cardene, Synalar, Synemol, Ticlid, Lidex, Nasalide

WYETH-AYERST

Program Name:	Wyeth Indigent Patient Program
Phone:	1-800-568-9938
Address:	Professional Services 150-A3
	Indigent Patient Program
	Wyeth-Ayerst Laboratories
	P.O. Box 8299
	Philadelphia, PA 19101-8299
Eligibility:	Ineligible for third-party reimbursement
Requirements:	Complete form
	Two-month supply sent to physician's office
Medications:	Phospholine Iodide
	Diamox sequels

	Diamox tablets
	Neptazane
Other Meds:	All manufactured products except controlled substances, injectables, and oral contraceptives
Turnover:	Four to six weeks
Refill:	Resubmit paperwork after two months
Contact:	Audrey Ashby, Director of Public Relations
Other:	Can duplicate enrollment forms
	No calls from patients

INDEX

Index